Vascular Surgery
Made Easy®

System requirement:
- Operating System-Windows XP or above
- Web Browser–Internet Explorer 8 or above, Google Chrome, Mozilla Firefox and Safari
- Essential plugins–Java and Flash player
  - Facing problems in viewing content – it may be your system does not have java enabled.
  - If Videos don't show up – it may be the system requires Flash player or need to manage flash setting
  - You can test java and flash by using the links from the troubleshoot section of the CD/DVD.
  - Learn more about flash setting from the link in the troubleshoot section.

Accompanying CD/DVD ROM is playable only in Computer and not in DVD player.
CD/DVD has Autorun function–it may take few seconds to load on your computer. If it does not work for you, then follow the steps below to access the contents manually:
- Click on my computer
- Select the CD/DVD drive and click open/explore – this will show list of files in the CD/DVD
- Find and double click file – "launch.html".

■ DVD CONTENTS

DVD—1

DVD—2

DVD—3

Vascular Surgery
Made Easy®

Manohar B Kalbande
MBBS MS (Surg) MCh (CVTS) FACS (CVTS, USA) FICS (CVTS) FIACS (CVTS)
Reeve Bett`s Fellow (CVTS) Clinical Fellow in CVTS
(Manchester Royal Infirmary, UK) European Society for
Vascular Surgery Fellowship FAIMS FCCP LLB PGDMLS

Honorary Cardiovascular and Thoracic Surgeon
Department of Cardiovascular and Thoracic Surgery
Government Medical College and Hospital
Aurangabad, Maharashtra, India

Honorary Professor and Head
Department of Cardiovascular and Thoracic Surgery
Mahatma Gandhi Mission's Medical College
Aurangabad, Maharashtra, India

JAYPEE BROTHERS MEDICAL PUBLISHERS (P) LTD.
New Delhi • London • Philadelphia • Panama

Jaypee Brothers Medical Publishers (P) Ltd.

Headquarters

Jaypee Brothers Medical Publishers (P) Ltd.
4838/24, Ansari Road, Daryaganj
New Delhi 110 002, India
Phone: +91-11-43574357
Fax: +91-11-43574314
Email: jaypee@jaypeebrothers.com

Overseas Offices

J.P. Medical Ltd.
83, Victoria Street, London
SW1H 0HW (UK)
Phone: +44-2031708910
Fax: +02-03-0086180
Email: info@jpmedpub.com

Jaypee-Highlights Medical Publishers Inc.
City of Knowledge, Bld. 237, Clayton
Panama City, Panama
Phone: +507-301-0496
Fax: +507-301-0499
Email: cservice@jphmedical.com

Jaypee Brothers Medical Publishers (P) Ltd.
17/1-B Babar Road, Block-B, Shaymali
Mohammadpur, Dhaka-1207
Bangladesh
Mobile: +08801912003485
Email: jaypeedhaka@gmail.com

Jaypee Brothers Medical Publishers (P) Ltd.
Shorakhute, Kathmandu
Nepal
Phone: +00977-9841528578
Email: jaypee.nepal@gmail.com

Jaypee Brothers Medical Publishers Ltd.
The Bourse
111, South Independence Mall East
Suite 835, Philadelphia, PA 19106, USA
Phone: + 267-519-9789
Email: joe.rusko@jaypeebrothers.com

Website: www.jaypeebrothers.com
Website: www.jaypeedigital.com

© 2013, Jaypee Brothers Medical Publishers

Vascular Surgery Made Easy®

First Edition: **2013**

ISBN 978-93-5090-394-0

Printed at Sanat Printers, Kundli.

Dedicated to

*Lord Buddha as based on the principles of Buddhism
I have become a good human being
and
My parents Late Captain Balaji Kalbande and
Late Nitabai Kalbande who taught me the importance
of hard work, devotion and sincerity*

Preface

Specialty of vascular surgery is relatively young. I was appointed as the Head, Department of Cardiovascular and Thoracic Surgery, Government Medical College, Aurangabad, Maharashtra, India, in 1985. At that time, this center was the only one catering to the needs of vascular surgical patients coming from 8 to 10 districts and from adjacent states. All types of vascular diseases patients, such as inflammatory, traumatic, atherosclerotic, etc. were flowing. Initially, the results were not encouraging because facilities were meager. Only investigations in the form of X-ray and simple ultrasound were available. Fine sutures and instruments were not available. But with persistent efforts, lots of patients started availing beneficial results. Even saccular thoracic aneurysms, abdominal aortic aneurysms and occlusions were operated, whenever some grafts were donated by missionaries. The experience started getting accumulated. The Association of Vascular Surgeons of India was formed in 1994 and regular conferences were then organized. With the experience and knowledge of experts from India and abroad through lectures and presentations delivered in such conferences, I got lots of information and encouragement. So, I started to analyze my experience over more than 25 years. I had a strong desire to place this experience in the hands of my beloved students in the form of book. This opportunity was provided by M/s Jaypee Brothers Medical Publishers (P) Ltd., New Delhi, India, as a result, the first edition is ready to be placed in the hands of students. As this is a short book, meant for undergraduate and postgraduate students; for further details, they are requested to refer texbooks on vascular surgery. Still I am sure in day-to-day studies, this book will be definitely useful, which will give tremendous satisfaction.

Manohar B Kalbande

Acknowledgments

It was not easy to write a book on vascular surgery as my routine activities did not permit me sufficient time. Emergency and routine scheduled operations, daily teaching schedule, etc. demand lots of time. This task would have been impossible without the help of following persons.

Dr Kranti Mahajan, General and Vascular Surgeon, helped me in all operative cases. Dr Jiten Kulkarni, Plastic and Reconstructive Surgeon, was always available for tissue cover and microvascular anastomosis, which was compiled and presented in this book. Dr Pravin Suryawanshi, Professor and Head, Department of Surgery and Chief Executive Officer of Mahatma Gandhi Mission's Medical College, Aurangabad, Maharashtra, India, allowed me to use clinical material from the institute, whenever required. I am grateful to all these persons for helping me.

My sincere thanks are also due to Mr Vivek Dusane, Computer Consultant, who helped me to organize all the script, photographs and videos. Because of his hard work, the book is in the present shape.

I thank my family members for supporting me and working extra hours with me during the preparation of this book. Last but not least, I sincerely thank all my patients who had undergone the procedures, which are included in this book.

Contents

Introduction

For decades, cardiac and vascular specialties were combined as a broad specialty of cardiovascular surgery. Due to glamor and challenges in cardiac surgery, majority of the surgeons devoted their time and skill for cardiac surgery and less time was available for developing vascular surgery. Cardiac surgeon colleagues also did not have time to study in-depth vascular diseases. So their involvement in vascular surgery remained limited to application of their cardiac surgical skill to vascular surgery, but the concept about the vascular diseases was not clear. Hence, gradually general surgeons and some of the interested cardiac surgeons started studying the subject with full devotion of time and skill. This led to the development of vascular surgery as an independent specialty.

Vascular surgery is a specialty dealing with diseases of arteries, veins and lymphatics. As there is no medicine counterpart, such as cardiology for cardiac surgery and neurology for neurosurgery, vascular surgeon has to deal with both medical and surgical aspects of the diseases. Consequently, newer techniques have been developed of endovascular grafting for thoracic and abdominal aneurysms, which has proved to be patient-friendly. Molecular Biology and Genetic Engineering are making their impact in further development of the specialty. Duplex ultrasound imaging, CT angiography with 3D reconstruction, MR angiography, IVUS, etc. are the investigative modalities, which are proving very much helpful in diagnosis and follow-up of the patients.

The knowledge of vascular specialty is vast and volume of knowledge is being added regularly. Hence, it becomes impossible even for the comprehensive textbooks to accommodate the expanding knowledge and to update. The present book is meant to be a short book for learning fundamentals of vascular surgery, which should prove useful for medical and postgraduate students. For comprehensive knowledge, the students are advised to refer the textbooks. Video DVD of the most commonly performed procedures is being provided. I hope, this book will prove to be of great help to the students and make them interested in the vascular surgery as their career in future.

Investigations in Peripheral Vascular Disease: Radiology and Imaging

Abstract

Paraphernalia of imaging and radiological modalities are available for vascular work up. For emergency screening, even hand held Doppler is enough. If time permits and in chronic cases, duplex ultrasound scan is an excellent investigation. If revascularization is planned, CTA/DSA/MRA any of them will give adequate information, selection being based on individual patient's parameters. Standard contrast angiography is not required on regular basis.

The exact incidence of peripheral vascular disease (PVD) is difficult to calculate. Approximately 5% people above the age of 60 years suffer from PVD. The incidence definitely rises with associated risk factors like DM, HTN, ischemic heart disease, smoking, etc. In case of symptomatic patients, diagnosis is not an issue, but the imaging modality is helpful to assess the severity and to plan intervention. While in case of asymptomatic or mildly symptomatic patients diagnosis and planning conservative therapy both depend on assessment by different modalities available. They are divided in two broad categories:

1. Invasive
2. Noninvasive.

Following modalities are usually utilized.

Ankle Brachial Index (Fig. 1.1)

Ankle brachial index (ABI) is a bedside investigation done with the help of hand held Doppler. Patient should lie comfortably supine and relaxed. Using cuff around arm, brachial artery systolic blood pressure is measured. Similarly, systolic BP is measured on DPA and PTA at ankle. Higher of the two is accepted. By dividing ankle systolic pressure by brachial systolic pressure, ABI is obtained. Normal ABI is 1-1.1, ABI of 0.9 or less indicates PAD, <=0.6 indicates critical ischemia <=0.3 indicates likely major tissue loss. The ABI in multisegmental disease is lower than that in single level obstruction. It is higher

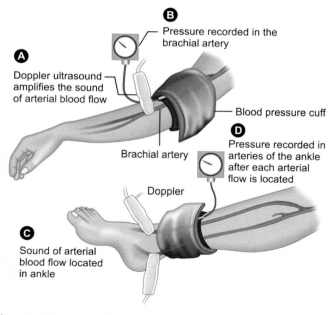

A Doppler ultrasound amplifies the sound of arterial blood flow

B Pressure recorded in the brachial artery

Blood pressure cuff

Brachial artery

D Pressure recorded in arteries of the ankle after each arterial flow is located

Doppler

C Sound of arterial blood flow located in ankle

Fig. 1.1: Ankle brachial index

in noncompressible/calcific arteries like in DM. The ABI can also be used in follow-up of patients operated or on conservative management. Hence, it is a very useful test in outpatient department.

Segmental Pressure Measurements

Ankle brachial index though is suggestive of obstruction in blood flow, it cannot localize the same. Using pneumatic cuffs at four sites: Upper thigh, above knee, around calf and ankle level, systolic pressures are measured on DP/PT. Gradient of $> = 30$ mm Hg is suggestive of obstruction in the intervening segment. This test result is affected by multilevel obstruction, small thigh size, proximal iliac artery obstruction, etc. Hence this test is replaced by other modalities as described later.

Plethysmography

Plethysmography is a test, based on measurement of changes in volume of limb. Segmental plethysmography is performed using mercury or indium strain gauge to record limb volume changes. Air is also commonly used to inflate thigh, calf and ankle cuffs to produce 65 mm Hg pressure and pulse volume tracings are recorded. Normal dicrotic notch rules out proximal segmental disease, but absence of the same is not diagnostic of obstructive PAD. Plethysmography of toes and fingers with tiny cuffs recording PVR indicates status of proximal arteries, which is also sensitive to vasospasm.

Transcutaneous pO$_2$

Transcutaneous pO$_2$ (TCpO$_2$) assessment which indicates status of tissue perfusion at various levels like foot, above and below patella, reference point being infraclavicular area. The value is affected by variables like cutaneous blood flow, metabolic activity, oxyhemoglobin dissociation and O_2 diffusion through tissues. The value is low when tissue perfusion is appreciably affected. Resting value is >= 55 mm Hg. It is not affected by calcified arteries like in DM. Value of 'zero' does not mean 'no perfusion', but it indicates total consumption of O_2 due to slow flow. Measurements can be made after exercise induced ischemia, leg dependency, after O_2 inhalation, etc. Though indicative of tissue perfusion, being costly equipment and as it does not indicate site of occlusion, it is not being used commonly.

Laser Doppler Velocitometry

Laser Doppler velocitometry is available in advanced set up and is not used routinely.

Hand Held Unidirectional Doppler

Hand held unidirectional Doppler is a light weight, portable screening machine very much useful in emergency situations. It can detect vascular occlusion, stenosis, and distal collateral flow. Vessel can be marked for precise exploration. After revascularization, distal flow and graft flow can be assessed on operation table. The result is operator dependent and detailed assessment is not possible. But it is inexpensive and can be repeated any number of times.

Duplex Ultrasound Scanning (Figs 1.2 and 1.3)

Ultrasound beam of certain frequency is thrown on moving blood particles, which is reflected by the same. This produces shift in Doppler frequency, which is appreciated and directly converted into flow velocity by automatic scanner. Duplex ultrasound scanning (DUS) provides information about vessel wall, blood flow with color images and velocity of flow thus

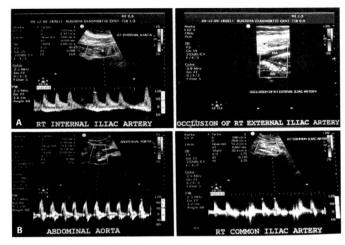

Figs 1.2A and B: Duplex ultrasound

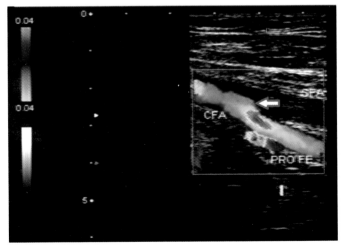

Fig. 1.3: Duplex ultrasound showing occlusion of external iliac artery

giving anatomical and physiological information. Addition of color flow signals is helpful in showing the direction of blood flow by red and green signals, thus differentiating between arterial and venous blood flow. Angle of Doppler probe should be <=60 degrees for best results. For superficial vessels 10-11 MHz and for deeper vessels 3-5 MHz probes are ideal. Though expensive and operator dependent, it provides excellent information about arterial and venous disorders. It can be quickly performed and repeated as required, portable machine can be used for bedside assessment in case the patient cannot be moved. Some of the centers are doing major revascularization on the basis of duplex ultrasound report, thus avoiding arteriography in emergency. The modality is very good for assessment of carotid, limb, mesenteric arteries and abdominal aorta.

Computed Tomographic Angiography (Fig. 1.4)

In present era, computed tomography facility is available even at remote places. Using the same computed tomographic angiography (CTA) can be performed for imaging vessels suspected to be affected. Initially intravenous contrast dye was used, which gave arterial images during recirculation phase. The images were not sharp and tissue overlapping further decreased sharpness. Using the intra-arterial contrast injection near the site of suspected disease excellent images can be obtained in different planes. Vessel wall details are also imaged and 3D reconstruction further increases diagnostic yield, which is very useful in planning surgery in AAA and carotid surgery, etc. The modality can give results quickly in emergency situations. There are some disadvantages like expensive equipment, need for trained people, complications related to ionic contrast injection, not suitable for renally compromised subjects and resolution not being comparable with invasive arteriography.

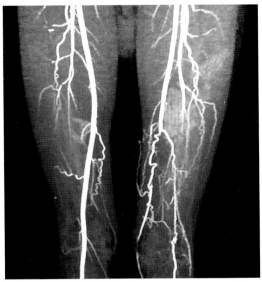

Fig. 1.4: CT angiography showing left femoral artery occlusion

Digital subtraction angiography is a modified imaging in which bone and soft tissue shadows overlapping vessels are removed and only vascular images can be studied. If required subtracted tissues can be superimposed to assess relation. Amount of contrast required is less and 3D reconstruction is possible. But the arterial wall cannot be seen.

Using CO_2 gas as contrast medium DSA is being done, which gives satisfactory images, though not comparable with standard arteriography. But it avoids fluid overload, helpful in cardiac patients and reactions to ionic contrast is also avoided. Using microcatheters for better CO_2 delivery, image quality can be improved.

Standard Invasive Arteriography (Fig. 1.5)

Standard invasive arteriography has been the gold standard for long time as the images it produces are excellent with which other imaging modalities are to be compared. It requires puncturing a palpable peripheral artery usually common femoral artery and introduction of catheter to inject contrast. The pictures are taken in rapid succession following the course of dye. It shows site of stenosis/obstruction, collaterals, distal run off/reformation of vessel, all these details being important to plan revascularization. It is to be used with caution in renally

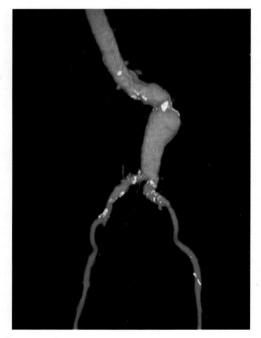

Fig. 1.5: Aortography

compromised patients. There may be reaction to dye, which can be avoided by using nonionic contrast. Local complications like hematoma, infection and distant ones like dissection, rupture/perforation, embolization, etc. must be carefully watched. Patient needs to be immobilized for 6-8 hours, which can be avoided by upper limb access if possible. Patient must be fully worked up for arteriography to avoid unforeseen complications.

Magnetic Resonance Imaging with Magnetic Resonance Angiography

It is a noninvasive modality of imaging. The subject is placed in a strong magnetic field, due to which hydrogen ions are rearranged while affecting flowing blood elements. It gives 3D images opacifying surrounding soft tissues along with blood vessels. Using nonionic contrast called gadolinium magnetic resonance angiography (MRA) can be done. It is a very good imaging modality for limb, extracranial arteries and for aorta and can be safely used in CRF patients. There is no exposure to radiation, hence it is safe. But it is very expensive, bulky machinery, patient may have phobia due to big gantry. Reporting takes time, hence it is not useful in emergency situation. It cannot be used when the subject has pacemaker, metallic prosthesis, metallic clips, dental prostheses, IVC filter, etc. in the body. Quality of images is not comparable with standard angiographic images. But no radiation, no dye reaction and reasonable resolution appear points in favor of its regular use.

Newer modalities like intravascular ultrasound (IVUS), angioscopy, nuclear scans, etc. are available in tertiary care and research institutes, which are going to find place in vascular armamentarium in future.

Acute Limb Ischemia

Introduction

Acute limb ischemia (ALI) is a challenging problem commonly faced by vascular surgeons in day-to-day practice. It is an emergency situation, which needs urgent attention and the outcome depends on the duration of ischemia, status of collateral circulation, time elapsed between admission and intervention and the completeness of revascularization.

Definition

Acute limb ischemia has been defined as a state of decreased perfusion of tissues of limb due to sudden cessation of blood flow occurring due to occlusion of axial artery (main artery of the limb) because of embolism or thrombosis. The duration extends from few minutes to 14 days.

Historical Aspects

History dates back to ancient times. In 1854, Virchow recognized sudden occlusion of artery by debris that was displaced from proximal remote site in the body and coined the term 'Embolus'. For long time conservative treatment was the only choice leading to amputation or death. McLean discovered

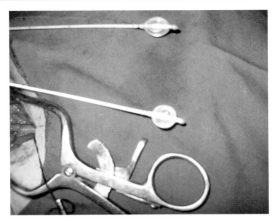

Fig. 2.1: Fogarty catheter

heparin and its clinical use started in 1932, which helped to prevent blood clotting, which was a great help in vascular interventions. The invention of balloon catheter by Thomas J Fogarty in 1963 revolutionized the management of ALI and produced gratifying results. Various types of balloon catheters later came into use (Fig. 2.1).

Etiology

There are four major categories:
1. Embolism
2. Thrombosis of native artery
3. Thrombosis of bypass graft
4. Vascular trauma.

Embolism

Embolism to peripheral arteries can occur due to:
a. Cardiac causes
b. Noncardiac causes.

Cardiac Causes

Emboli originate from heart in more than 90% cases secondary to various disorders as described below:

- Rheumatic heart disease involves cardiac valves and produces atrial fibrillation due to which stasis of blood occurs in left atrial appendage leading to thrombus formation. This can get dislodged and embolize during forceful heartbeat, to various locations including major limb arteries especially at bifurcation, which is called 'cardioarterial embolization'.
- After replacement of heart valves with prosthetic heart valves patients are put on lifelong anticoagulation. Due to inadequate anticoagulation or due to some mechanical valve related problem, thrombus may form around the valve and may get dislodged.
- After acute myocardial infarction, raw area may be created on endocardial surface of left ventricle, which becomes the site for thrombosis. It may embolize to periphery.
- Vegetations may form on native normal or diseased valve. In drug addicts due to repeated intravenous injections, vegetation may form on tricuspid valve. There may occur cardiac tumor like atrial myxoma which is friable. All these may produce arterial embolism.
- Intracardiac gadgets, such as pacemaker leads, implantable cardioversion device, etc. may be the site for thrombus formation and subsequent embolization.

Noncardiac Causes

- *Arterioarterial embolism:* Proximal major artery or aorta may be affected by atherosclerosis. The vulnerable plaque may rupture and thrombus may form on exposed plaque, which subsequently produces distal embolism after dislodgement.
- Primary or secondary malignant tumor may invade adjacent major artery producing intravascular extension. This

portion may get detached and produce distal embolism.

- Popliteal artery aneurysm is a common lesion in younger patients. It may get thrombosed and produce distal embolism.
- In recent years, interventions by the cardiologists are on the rise. Open heart operation also requires cannulation of major arteries and aorta. Invasive blood pressure monitoring in intensive care unit and in operation theater also requires inserting catheter in peripheral artery. All these gadgets may accidentally break and produce embolization.
- *Cryptogenic emboli:* In 5-10% cases of peripheral embolism source of embolism cannot be detected, which is put under cryptogenic embolism category.

Thrombosis of Native Artery

Atherosclerotic plaque may produce arterial stenosis, which gets totally occluded on thrombus formation on its exposed raw surface. Again occlusive thrombus formation may occur on a stenotic lesion, which may be produced by variety of disorders, such as inflammatory arteritis, arteritis in Takayasu's disease, nonspecific aortoarteritis, thromboangiitis obliterans. Thrombosis may occur at the site of popliteal artery aneurysm. Rarely, the popliteal artery entrapment syndrome, adventitial cystic disease of popliteal artery may be responsible for initiation of thrombosis. In normal native artery thrombosis may occur due to underlying hypercoagulable state induced by hyperhomocysteinemia, deficiency of protein C and S, antithrombin III, antiphospholipid antibody syndrome, etc. Sometimes, in rural area, tight tourniquet is applied by illiterate persons or by village quack to treat limb pain, snake bite or insect bite, which has been seen to produce circumferential injury including arterial and venous thrombosis as well as nerve injury, which is a ghastly injury in an otherwise totally preventable scenario.

Thrombosis of Bypass Graft (Figs 2.2 and 2.3)

In developed countries and also in developing countries, tertiary referral centers revascularization using either artificial graft or autologous saphenous vein is being performed on regular basis. Hence, occlusion of such a bypass graft in postoperative period has become one of the most common

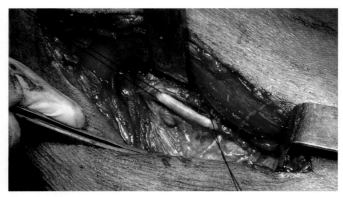

Fig. 2.2: Popliteal artery graft

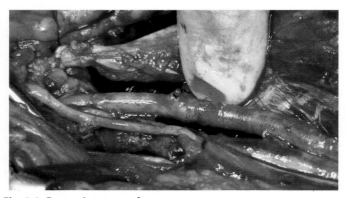

Fig. 2.3: Femoral artery graft

causes responsible for acute limb ischemia. Prosthetic graft may get occluded at anastomosis site usually distal, due to intimal hyperplasia. Vein graft may get occluded due to either retained valve in *in situ* graft or at stenotic segment in vein. If distal run off is not good, whole graft may get thrombosed.

Vascular Trauma (Figs 2.4 and 2.5)

Acute limb ischemia due to arterial injury is also common due to increased number of vehicular accidents. This has been dealt with separately in the chapter on Vascular Trauma.

Pathophysiology

Peripheral emboli lodge at the site of arterial bifurcation, such as abdominal aortic bifurcation, division of common femoral, popliteal, brachial arteries. In majority, around 70-80%

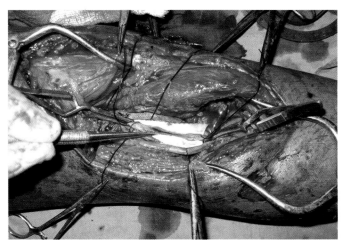

Fig. 2.4: Popliteal artery tear

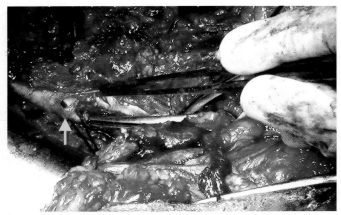

Fig. 2.5: Femoral artery tear

cases main or axial artery supplying the limb is occluded. In thrombosis, occlusion occurs at the site of stenosis. Changes secondary to hypoperfusion of the tissues beyond the site of occlusion start immediately. If there are pre-existing collaterals or there is sufficient time for the development of collaterals, significant changes may not occur. If the collateral vessels are not recruited or if the thrombus extends proximal and distal to the site of thrombus occluding collaterals, the ischemia worsens. Major thrombus may get fragmented and produce distal embolization. Due to ischemia, accumulation of toxic elements, such as free oxygen radicals, which produce all the damage. Severity of ischemic damage depends on type of tissue and its metabolic demand. Peripheral nerves are most sensitive and are damaged early, whereas the muscles can sustain ischemia for 4-6 hours. Subcutaneous tissue and skin are affected last.

Free radicals damage endothelial cell lining of arterioles, capillaries and venules, which become edematous and as a result the lumen gets occluded. Therefore, even if the circulation is restored after some time interval by revascularization, perfusion does not improve. So, there is no clinical improvement termed as 'no reflow phenomenon'. Due to increased capillary permeability protein and fluid leak into extravascular space producing edema and increase in hydrodynamic pressure. This may increase to an extent, which interferes with a venous drainage. Further rise in hydrodynamic pressure interferes with a arterial circulation and worsens the ischemia. Muscles become massively swollen due to increase in tissue pressure. When the muscles cannot swell further in the rigid fascial compartment ischemia worsens. This is called 'compartment syndrome'. Hence, release of this tension on muscles becomes vital in addition to revascularization.

Differences Between Embolism and Thrombosis (Table 2.1)

Table 2.1: Differences between embolism and thrombosis

	Embolism	**Thrombosis**
Onset	Acute	Not so
History of previous embolism	+	–
Source of embolism	+	–
Intermittent claudication	–	+
Proximal and contralateral pulse	+	May be absent
Ischemic changes	Marked	Less marked
Duplex scan	Normal in un-affected limb	Diffuse disease
Angiography	Sharp cut off	Tapered, irregular cut off
	Minimal disease	Diffuse disease
	Scanty collaterals	Good collaterals

Clinical Features (Table 2.1)

Presentation of ALI differs in embolism and thrombosis. In case of embolism, there is sudden onset of symptoms, whereas in case of thrombosis symptoms may be insidious due to pre-existing collaterals. Classical cardinal features of ALI are described by 6 P's used as mnemonics:

Pain	Pallor	Pulselessness
Paresthesia	Paralysis	Poikilothermia

Pain is of sudden onset in embolism, severe and continuous in nature. Pain if not continuous, may be elicited by passive movement of extremity. Duration, location, intensity, sudden onset and change over time must all be noted carefully. Previously palpable pulse is not felt. Temperature of the limb is reduced. Sensory disturbances, such as tingling, numbness may occur. In advanced ischemia, there may be total sensory loss. Later in the course of the disease, there may be motor nerve damage and ischemic damage to muscles leading to paralysis, which indicates quite a delayed status.

In the history of past illness, history of previous embolism and intermittent claudication should be enquired. History of smoking, diabetes mellitus, heart disease, hypercoagulable state, etc. must be enquired as these increase mortality.

In order to have uniformity, the extent of ALI has been classified by Society for Cardiovascular Surgery [SCS] Committee based on Rutherford criteria into three main classes:

Class I: Viable—The limb is viable without therapeutic intervention. There is no motor and sensory deficit. Doppler flow signals are clearly audible.

Class IIA: Marginally threatened—There are signs of critical ischemia with numbness, paresthesia or limited digital sensory loss and no arterial flow signals. Limb needs revascularization early.

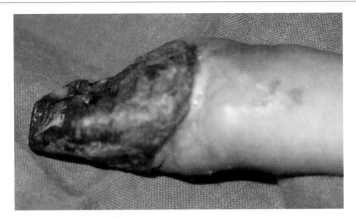

Fig. 2.6: Gangrene of hand

Class IIB: Immediately threatened—IIA + persistent ischemic pain, greater sensory loss and motor deficit. Limb needs urgent revascularization for salvage.

Class III: Irreversible—Profuse anesthesia and paralysis of the limb. Not salvageable (Fig. 2.6).

Diagnosis

Diagnosis of ALI is mostly clinical, based on the features described above. Measurement of Ankle Brachial Index (ABI) is a helpful parameter. The ABI below 0.4 indicates severe ischemia. Hand held Doppler is good enough to diagnose arterial occlusion, distal collateral flow if any, associated deep venous thrombosis. If time permits get quick duplex scan, which can be of great help as it gives better idea about site and type of occlusion, status of proximal and distal circulation. In not so emergency cases there could be a chance for CT angiography or MR angiography.

Treatment

Once the diagnosis is established, ECG and chest X-ray are done and blood sample is withdrawn for routine investigations. Then intravenous bolus of injection heparin 100 units/kg body weight is given. Immediate revascularization is necessary for limb salvage, to avoid morbidity and mortality, which are dependent on duration of ischemia, the speed of revascularization and its completeness. Modality of treatment does not depend upon duration of ischemia, but on the condition of limb.

Two modalities of treatment are available:
1. Surgical revascularization
2. Endovascular therapy

Generally speaking surgery is preferred in embolism involving proximal limb artery with ALI and in good risk patients, while endovascular therapy is preferred in distal thrombotic occlusion with subacute ischemia. General plan of treatment is usually as follows:

Class I and IIA: The first option is anticoagulation. There is usually time for duplex scan and angiographic evaluation and for evaluation of comorbid conditions like coronary artery disease.

Class IIB: Emergency surgery.

Class III: Usually amputation.

Surgical Revascularization (Figs 2.7 and 2.8; 2.1)

It is the treatment of choice for acute embolism and acute thrombosis of bypass graft or of native artery. It is done preferably under local anesthesia with a standby anesthetist, under regional anesthesia or under spinal anesthesia. Using appropriate size Fogarty balloon catheter embolus is retrieved. If there is distal embolus or back flow is not satisfactory or intraoperative angiography shows residual embolus, intra-arterial thrombolysis is done with urokinase 2.5 Lac units

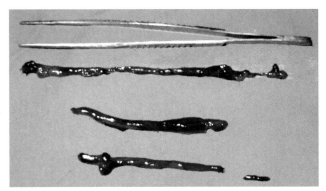

Fig. 2.7: Acute thrombus removed

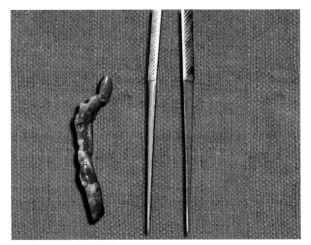

Fig. 2.8: Organized thrombus

infused over 30 minutes. It produces good result and palpable pulse. But after thrombolysis limb edema usually occurs due to reperfusion which subsides gradually.

Short segment thrombotic occlusion is treated with endarterectomy and removal of thrombus by dissection. Long segment occlusion is treated by bypass grafting. Conduit of choice for above knee bypass is polytetrafluoroethylene [PTFE] graft and reversed great saphenous vein for below knee bypass. In case of occluded venous bypass graft, revision with fresh vein graft is indicated. Occasionally long segment thrombus from major proximal artery can be removed by Fogarty adherent clot retrieval catheter by arteriotomy and bypass can be avoided.

In patients presenting with delayed ischemia and with compartment syndrome, fasciotomy must be done to release the pressure on the muscles.

Mortality is higher in surgically treated patients due to complications associated with severe ischemia and due to associated comorbid conditions, such as coronary artery disease, myocardial infarction, arrhythmia, pneumonia, chronic renal failure, etc.

Endovascular Therapy (Fig. 2.9)

It utilizes plasminogen activator, such as urokinase, reteplase or alteplase. Urokinase is the most commonly used agent being cheap and easily available. Reteplase produces rapid lysis but is expensive. Using multihole catheter placed in the thrombus usually 2.5 Lac unit bolus is given followed by 4000 units per minute for 4 hours, then 2000 units per minute until complete lysis occurs as confirmed by check angiography.

Advantages of thrombolytic therapy: Clot dissolution occurs predictably and under angiographic control. Underlying lesion, such as aneurysm is revealed. There is reduced need for surgical intervention, with equal limb salvage rate.

Disadvantages: Suitable for early, i.e. for class I and IIA patients, prolonged duration of therapy, local and remote hemorrhagic complications do occur. It is contraindicated in recent major

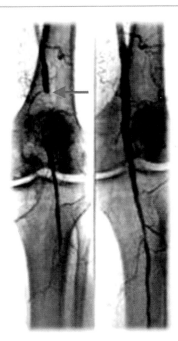

Fig. 2.9: Popliteal artery thrombolysis

bleed and stroke, in recent major surgery and trauma, in recent major gastrointestinal bleed. It is relatively contraindicated in pregnancy, severe hypertension, coagulation abnormality, etc.

Mechanical Thrombectomy Devices

These devices have become available and are being used increasingly over past few years. Some devices use hydrodynamic, rheolytic forces, while others use rotational motion. The fragmented thrombi are sucked out. Still thrombolysis is required after mechanical thrombectomy for better distal clearance.

Comparison of thrombolytic therapy with surgery failed to establish superiority of the former in STILE, TOPAS trials. Hence, the choice of treatment still remains subjective. Drugs requiring shorter duration with less bleeding complications for thrombolysis aided by mechanical devices could be used more frequently in future.

Complications of Revascularization for ALI

A. Reperfusion syndrome occurs due to re-establishment of blood flow to acutely ischemic limb, which can cause myoglobinemia, myoglobinuria, acute tubular necrosis, metabolic acidosis, hyperkalemia, cardiac arrhythmias, etc. These complications could be life threatening.

B. Due to capillary edema peripheral tissue perfusion may not improve despite axial artery clearance, termed as 'no reflow phenomenon'.

C. Compartment syndrome has already been described. If fasciotomy is not performed early Volkmann`s ischemic contracture or limb loss may occur. After fasciotomy, the bleeding and infection are likely complications.

Result

Mortality of 10-20% and limb salvage rate in the range of 70-90% has been shown in many studies. Mortality is usually due to cardiac or renal causes.

Chronic Lower
Limb Ischemia

Prevalence

Chronic lower limb ischemia is one of the most common problems as vascular surgeon has to face in day-to-day practice. Patient may present with a spectrum of clinical picture from being totally asymptomatic to having intermittent claudication or may have tissue necrosis with rest pain which is a sign of critical limb ischemia. It is more common in males and about 10% patients affected are more than 70 years of age. About 50% have multisegmental disease. About 1 in 4 patients develop progressive symptoms and revascularization is required in approximately 20% patients at 10 years. Amputation rate is 1-7% at 5-10 years. With continued smoking and uncontrolled diabetes mellitus, disease progresses fast. Diabetic patients are >15 times more likely to have amputation than nondiabetic patients. Mortality rate in claudicants is 50% at 5 years and 70% for critical ischemia patients. High mortality rate is associated with cardiac problems.

Definitions

Critical limb ischemia (CLI): It has been defined by Trans Atlantic inter Society Consensus (TASC) conference as persistent, recurring ischemic rest pain requiring opiate analgesia for at least 2 weeks, ulceration or gangrene of the toes or foot (Fig. 3.1), having ankle systolic pressure of 50 mm Hg or less, toe systolic pressure of 30 mm Hg or less. Most but not all the subjects with rest pain or tissue necrosis have limb loss. About 30% patients with CLI have significant coronary artery disease and about 30% have carotid stenosis of more than 50%.

Intermittent claudication (IC): It is the lower extremity muscular pain felt in calf muscles, less frequently in thighs and buttocks, induced by exercise and relieved with short periods of rest and is caused by inadequate increase in muscle blood flow on demand due to proximal arterial obstruction.

Risk Factors

Smoking

Tobacco consumption is the most important risk factor for the peripheral arterial disease (PAD). Smokers are four times more prone to develop PAD as compared to nonsmokers. More than 80% subjects with IC have history of smoking. Exact underlying

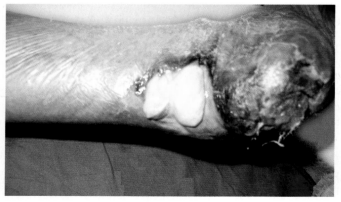

Fig. 3.1: Ischemic ulcers—leg and heel

mechanism is controversial and not well-understood. It appears that there are multiple factors acting together like alteration of vascular endothelium, prostaglandin mechanism, neutrophil activation, platelet activation, altered lipid metabolism, blood viscosity, coagulation, etc. Lower intake of nutrients like betacarotene, vitamin C may lead to increased oxidation of fatty acids and atherogenicity of low density lipoprotein (LDL) cholesterol. Continued smoking leads to increased amputation rate and graft failure and total cessation of smoking produces good clinical improvement.

Diabetes Mellitus

Diabetes mellitus is a strong risk factor in development of PAD. Progression of atherosclerosis is more rapid and involvement of infrainguinal proximal arteries is more common. Risk of amputation is 15-20 times more than in nondiabetics.

Hypertension

Hypertension is more common in PAD patients and may have synergistic effect with smoking by increasing movement of nicotine across the endothelial cell membrane.

Hyperlipidemia

Increased LDL and triglycerides are associated with increased cardiovascular and cerebrovascular morbidity and is a common abnormality in PAD patients. Control of lipids reduces need for revascularization and reduces cardiac mortality.

Hyperhomocysteinemia

Hyperhomocysteinemia is associated with increased risk of PAD. It is detrimental to vascular endothelium, increases auto-oxidation of LDL cholesterol, enhances smooth muscle cell proliferation and accelerates atherosclerosis. But its reduction with folic acid and B-complex has not shown regression of atherosclerosis.

Other Factors

Hypercoagulable state, increased factors VIII, XIII, plasminogen, sedentary lifestyle, excessive alcohol consumption, etc. may be responsible as contributory factors for development of PAD.

Etiology

a. Atherosclerosis is the single most important cause for occlusive PAD, which is hastened by the risk factors as mentioned earlier.
b. Thromboangiitis obliterans
c. Vasculitis
d. Arterial trauma
   Entities b, c, d are described in details in respective chapters separately.
e. *Popliteal artery entrapment syndrome:* More than 50% patients younger than 50 years with history of IC have popliteal artery entrapment syndrome. It is often bilateral and occurs due to compression by muscle or tendinous bands. Passive dorsiflexion of foot or active plantar flexion against resistance may obliterate pedal pulses or may produce bruit on popliteal artery.
f. *Adventitial cystic disease:* It affects male in 15:1 ratio, in 3rd and 4th decade of life. Popliteal, femoral, external iliac and other arteries which are in proximity of joints are affected. There is a cystic clear mucinous fluid collection in the adventitial layer of arteries. Due to proximity of joints, it has been suggested that during embryological development mucin secreting cells derived from the mesenchyme of the adjacent joints are included in the adventitia of the arteries.

g. *Other nonatherosclerotic causes:* Aortic coarctation, Takayasu's arteritis, radiation injury, popliteal aneurysm, arterial fibrodysplasia, pseudoxanthoma elasticum, persistent sciatic artery, iliac syndrome of the cyclists, primary vascular tumors, etc.

Pathophysiology

Although pathophysiology of atherosclerosis is not fully understood, it appears to be a dynamic process. Changes occurring in proximal large vessels produce occlusion or stenosis, but changes also occur at microvascular level which should be understood.

- *Microvascular changes:* Atheromatous plaque develops in three stages.
    - *Early lesion:* Lipid laden foam cells are deposited in the intima, which produce yellow streaks and appear as fatty streaks on the intima.
    - Connective tissue elements and smooth muscle cells are deposited over fatty streaks producing fibrous cap. This may cause partial or complete occlusion of the arterial lumen.
    - Complications may occur in fibrous plaque like ulceration, calcification and hemorrhage.

    Ulceration exposes underlying plaque which is highly thrombogenic to flowing blood which leads to platelet activation and deposition. Rupture of plaque or hemorrhage underneath may produce partial or total cessation of blood flow producing critical limb ischemia (myocardial infarction in heart and stroke in brain). In addition, peripheral embolization of the material may occur producing small arterial occlusion and ischemic pain. Chronic occlusion produces opening of collateral vessels which are pre-existing and supply blood beyond the level of occlusion. Collateral anastomosis between profunda femoris and geniculate arteries around knee joint is atypical example of collateral circulation. This is a feature of chronic lower limb ischemia.

- *Microcirculation:* It consists of arterioles, capillaries, venules, interstitium and lymphatics. In chronic occlusion, there is decreased tissue perfusion, which stimulates elements of microcirculation for compensatory changes, the first one being vasodilatation. Consequently, cells take more time to travel, hence greater interaction with endothelium and more plasma viscosity. This leads to RBC clumping and release of ADP which promotes platelet aggregation. Vasoactive substances are released which damage vascular endothelium, produce endothelial swelling and increased permeability. This further reduces tissue nutrition. Maldistribution of blood flow reduces skin blood flow and nutrition making it more prone to injury.

Clinical Features

There is a spectrum of clinical features, the severity has been defined by Fontaine's classification as follows:
- *Stage 1:* Asymptomatic
- *Stage 2:* Intermittent claudication limiting lifestyle
- *Stage 3:* Ischemic rest pain
- *Stage 4:* Tissue necrosis (ulcer, gangrene) due to ischemia
  Intermittent claudication has already been defined earlier. For every patient of IC, there could be three more without any symptom. With adequate collaterals and partial arterial occlusion, the same status may be maintained for a long time. Progression of ischemia produces rest pain, intermittent claudication over shorter distance, ulcer or gangrene. Proximal aortoiliac obstruction produces IC, while infrainguinal occlusion produces tissue necrosis. Younger patients may experience impotence with aortoiliac disease. Distal embolization from aortoiliac plaque may produce ischemia of toes called 'blue toe syndrome'.

Clinical Examination

It must include palpation of all peripheral pulses and graded as follows:

3- Hyperdynamic bounding/ collapsing pulse

2- Normal

1- Decreased pulse volume

0- Absent pulse.

Wasting of muscles, shiny hairless ischemic skin, ulcer location (arterial ulcers more common on forefoot and toes, venous ulcers on medial malleolus) should be noted. Record blood pressure and ankle brachial index. Examine cardiovascular system for possible ischemic heart disease and arrhythmias, respiratory system for COPD and central nervous system for carotid arterial disease.

In younger patients without atherosclerosis risk, one must suspect hyperhomocysteinemia, popliteal artery entrapment and aneurysm.

Differential Diagnosis

Root compression due to herniated disk or osteophyte, hip arthritis, diabetic neuropathy must be differentiated from chronic atherosclerotic ischemia, which sometimes is really difficult.

Investigations

   i. Hb, CBC, platelets

  ii. BS- F/ PP

 iii. Renal function tests

 iv. Lipid profile

  v. Urinalysis

 vi. Serum homocysteine

vii. Tests for hypercoagulability in younger patients

viii. ECG in elderly patient

 ix. Carotid Doppler study desirable

    x. Duplex ultrasound scan with sensitivity of 92% and specificity of 98% is an ideal screening mode for chronic arterial occlusion. It identifies site, length of occlusion, proximal and distal patency. It is not very suitable for distal most arteries. But it is beneficial in many ways as it is cheap, can be repeated, is available at many peripheral centers and patient's safety is not compromised.

    xi. Computed tomographic angiography (CTA) is advised if vascular intervention is planned. The CTA can image aortoiliac, visceral, crural and pedal arteries nicely, but contrast related morbidity and mortality must be remembered. If possible contrast enhanced conventional angiography should be done, which is a gold standard.

    xii. *MRI with MRA:* Gadolinium enhanced MRA is very useful diagnostic modality in renally compromised patients to image arterial occlusion, but the equipment is costly, not easily available at peripheral places, takes time to give report, cannot be done in patients having metal implants and some patients may have claustrophobia to heavy gantry of MRI.

Medical Management

a. Smoking cessation is the mainstay of treatment.

b. Ischemic heart disease to be treated with antianginal drugs, statins, antiplatelet drugs, ACE inhibitors, antiarrhythmic drugs, etc.

c. Hypertension to be treated preferably with ACE inhibitor and beta-blocker.

d. Diabetes mellitus to be treated with injection insulin and oral hypoglycemic drugs as per requirement.

e. Hyperlipidemia to be treated with statins to reduce total cholesterol below 200 mg/dl and LDL cholesterol below 100 mg/dl.

f. Hyperhomocysteinemia: To be treated with folic acid and vitamin B complex.

g. Exercise program to increase intermittent claudication distance.

Drug Therapy for Intermittent Claudication

Cilostazol: It is PDE III inhibitor, which increases cyclic AMP, produces vasodilatation, has antiplatelet effect and modifies plasma proteins. Ideal dose is 100 mg BID and can be given for prolonged duration. In older patients as maintenance 50 mg BID dose is sufficient. Side effects like headache, diarrhea, palpitation force about 15% patients to stop therapy. Major contraindication is congestive heart failure.

Pentoxifylline: It was being used for long time before cilostazol. Currently widespread use of it is not supported. Use of pentoxifylline did not show any improvement over placebo in controlled studies.

Naftidrofuryl: It is serotonin antagonist acts over aerobic metabolism in oxygen deprived tissues. It also decreases platelet aggregation. It is popular in Europe but not approved in the USA.

Blufomedil: It reduces alpha 1-2 mediated vasoconstriction, decreases platelet aggregation. Near about 40% improvement in walking distance has been observed. It is also being used in Europe, but not approved in the USA.

Carnitine: It augments metabolism in the ischemic muscle by converting acetyl-CoA into free CoA and acetyl carnitine, improving fatty acid metabolism. Hence, 50-60% improvement occurs in maximum walking distance thereby significantly improving quality of life.

Prostaglandins: Relax smooth muscles, reduce platelet aggregation and suppress smooth muscle cell proliferation.

But uniform encouraging results have not been obtained. Side effects like headache, palpitation, diarrhea, force more than 50% patients to stop the therapy. It is also not cost effective for poor patients.

Vascular endothelial growth factor (VEGF): It promotes neoangiogenesis, more collaterals develop. Initial results show healing of ischemic ulcers and relief of pain, but further results must be awaited.

L-arginine: Nitric oxide NO maintains normal endothelial function, produces vasodilatation, reduces platelet aggregation. It has been found to be inhibited in PAD. L-arginine is dietary supplement precursor of endogenous NO. It may prove to be of help in the treatment of PAD.

Surgical Revascularization

Most common site of atherosclerotic occlusion is distal abdominal aorta near bifurcation extending into common iliac arteries. Depending upon the distribution of disease, there are three types:

Type I: Localized disease confined to distal abdominal aorta and common iliac arteries.

Type II: More widespread intra-abdominal disease than type I.

Type III: Multilevel disease with infrainguinal occlusive disease.

Aortoiliac endarterectomy: It is possible for type I disease. It is done by laparotomy and direct incision over aorta followed by dissection and removal of thrombus from aortoiliac bifurcation. As it avoids use of artificial graft, cost of the procedure is less and complication like infection can be avoided. But it is a major procedure and rethrombosis rate is high. Hence, it is not being used commonly (Fig. 3.2).

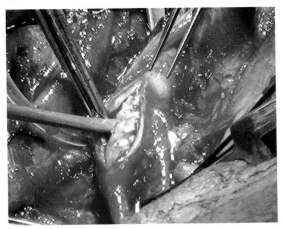

Fig. 3.2: Common femoral artery thrombus

Aortobifemoral bypass: By laparotomy aortic bifurcation is exposed and common femoral arteries are exposed in groin. Dacron graft of Y shape and of different sizes, e.g. 12 × 6, 14 × 7 mm, etc. are available. Adequate size graft is selected. Proximal end of the graft is sutures to infrarenal disease free aorta in end to side fashion and distal limbs are sutured to respective CFA in groin in end to side fashion.

Infrainguinal bypass: Appropriate bypass procedure is done from proximal normal artery to distal patent vessel beyond the obstruction. Choice of bypass conduit is either polytetrafluoroethylene (PTFE) graft or autologous reversed saphenous vein in above knee location, but for below knee bypass, reversed or *in situ* saphenous vein is a must, as the patency of artificial graft is low in below knee position. Good run off in distal vessel after bypass is a must for long-term patency (Figs 3.3 to 3.5).

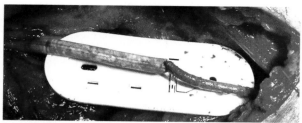

Fig. 3.3: CFA-PTA composite graft

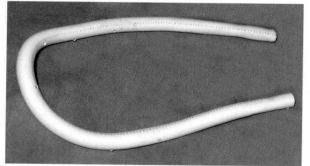

Fig. 3.4: A 6 mm PTFE graft

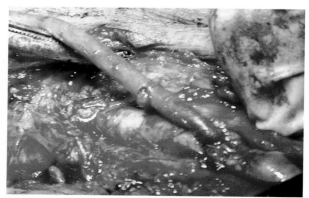

Fig. 3.5: Reversed saphenous vein graft to PTA

Extra-anatomical bypass: In high-risk surgical patients and in subjects having hostile abdomen or infected intra-abdominal graft, extra-anatomical graft like axillofemoral or femorofemoral can be carried out in selected patients.

Endovascular Intervention

Percutaneous transluminal angioplasty (PTA) is a technique of dilatation of focal stenosis using a balloon. Lesion suitable for PTA should be localized stenosis preferably of less than 5 cm long and should be stenosis than total occlusion involving aorta, iliac arteries or proximal femoral arteries.

Stent placement can be done for dissection or residual stenosis after PTA (Figs 3.6 and 3.7). It does not allow the opened lumen to close again immediately. It is possible to combine stenting with bypass procedure in some difficult

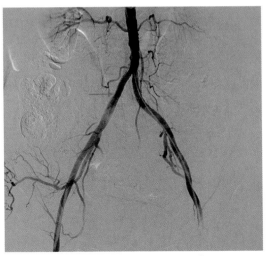

Fig. 3.6: Aortography showing RT CIA post stenting

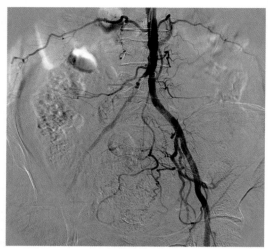

Fig. 3.7: Aortography showing RT CIA occlusion

situations or in multisegmental disease, what is called 'hybrid procedure'. Overall patency of infrapopliteal PTA and stent is inferior to bypass procedure using autologous vein in long-term follow-up.

Endovascular stent graft has become available in various sizes for type I disease and is being successfully inserted at selected centers with low morbidity. But the cost of the stented graft is very high and the expertise is not available at many centers. But in future, when the cost comes down and the experience accumulates, it is likely to become a commonly performed procedure being patient-friendly with low morbidity.

Thus with availability of many drugs, bypass and endovascular interventions it is definitely possible to relieve ischemic pain of many who are victims of chronic lower limb ischemia.

chapter 4

Thromboangiitis Obliterans/Buerger's Disease

History

Von Winiwater in 1879 studied vessels in amputated limb of an old man, having pain in the limb for 12 years. He found thrombosis, fibrosis and intimal proliferation. In 1908, Leo Buerger studied 11 amputated limbs of smokers. He suggested occurrence of endarteritis, and endophlebitis, which he said was different from atherosclerosis. He named it as thromboangiitis obliterans (TAO).

Definition

The TAO is nonatherosclerotic, segmental, inflammatory disease affecting small-and medium-sized arteries and veins mostly in extremities. It occurs in smokers and is different from vasculitis.

Incidence

It is more common in males than females, though the incidence in females is rising. It occurs only in smokers. It involves lower extremity more commonly than the upper one. Other arteries are also rarely involved. It is more common in people of low socioeconomic group. It has worldwide distribution, incidence in Japan being 5 per lac population. There is high incidence in Indian bidi smokers.

Etiology

Though TAO is thought to be a type of vasculitis, it is different from it as:

i. Thrombus is highly cellular, internal elastic lamina is preserved.

ii. Inflammatory parameters, such as ESR, CRP are not elevated.

iii. Autoantibodies, such as RA factor, ANA, etc. are normal or negative.

Smoking

Though etiology of TAO is not clear, there is extremely strong association of heavy tobacco consumption and TAO. There is very high incidence amongst Indian heavy bidi smokers (unprocessed tobacco wrapped in leaves) belonging to low socioeconomic strata as mentioned earlier. There has not been a well-documented TAO case in nonsmoker. There could be some hypersensitive response to tobacco ingredients producing inflammatory response. But worldwide only a small number of smokers develop TAO, suggesting thereby that there could be other factors playing role in etiology.

Genetic Factors

Genetic factors could play some role in making smokers prone for developing disease. At present, there is no clear information about this.

Hypercoagulability

Various factors related to platelets, coagulation mechanism, hyperhomocysteinemia, etc. have been incriminated, but further studies are required.

Endothelial Dysfunction

Acetylcholine causes endothelium dependent and sodium nitroprusside endothelium independent vasodilatation. Using them, it has been shown that endothelium dependent vasodilatation is impaired in TAO patients, both in affected and nonaffected limbs. So vasoconstriction may be more pronounced in them.

Immunological Mechanisms

Data from various publications has suggested that immunological activation may be in part important pathogenetic factor. T cell mediated cellular immunity and B cell mediated humoral immunity may produce endarteritis.

In summary, etiology of TAO though uncertain, tobacco consumption plays definite role, whereas other factors, such as hyper-coagulation, immunological factors, endothelial dysfunction and genetic predisposition could play some role.

Pathology

Pathological findings in TAO depend on the chronological age of the disease. In chronic cases, there may not be any diagnostic feature. Histopathology is typically seen in an acute case with episode of thrombophlebitis. There is occlusive thrombus in the lumen polymorphs infiltrating in it. Cellular infiltrate is more in the thrombus than in the wall. In later stages, thrombus gets organized and recanalized with a perivascular fibrosis. Internal elastic lamina remains intact. There is typically segmental vessel involvement. In older individuals atherosclerotic changes may also be present. Apart from common involvement of limb arteries, visceral, coronary, carotid vessels may be rarely involved.

Clinical Features

It typically occurs in young, adult male, who is a smoker or consumes tobacco in any form, the age group being 40-45 years. It is less common in females (77:23). Only lower limb involvement occurs in 75% cases, combined upper and lower limbs in 20% and isolated upper limb in 5% approximately. Involvement of other vessels is quite rare as commented earlier.

Following symptoms occur in descending order. Rest pain is the most common. Ischemic ulcers can occur in digits (Figs 4.1 and 4.2). Intermittent claudication and recurrent migratory thrombophlebitis may occur in some cases, especially in early course of the disease. Some patients have features of vasculitis (Raynaud's phenomenon) and sensory changes may

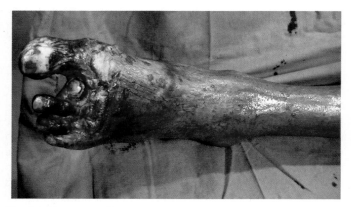

Fig. 4.1: Gangrene of toes

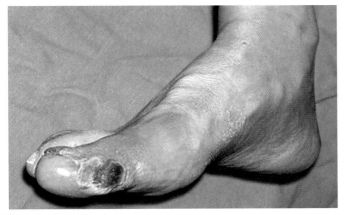

Fig. 4.2: Great toe ulcer

be seen in digits. Even in lower limb TAO, Allen's test may be positive (suggestive of vascular compromise in upper limb), which may indicate possibility of multiple limb involvement. Early cases may have foot and arch claudication, which may be confused with an orthopedic ailment and hence diagnosis and treatment may be delayed.

Shinoya's diagnostic criteria for TAO:

- Onset < 50 years of age
- History of smoking
- Involvement of infrapopliteal arteries
- Upper limb involvement does occur
- Migrating superficial thrombophlebitis
- Absent atherosclerotic risk factors except for smoking.

Investigations

There is no diagnostic test for TAO. Following tests are advised:

1. Hb for anemia and CBC for treatment for infection if any.
2. ESR, CRP should be normal.

3. BSL for DM, lipid profile for better atherosclerotic/ lipid management.

4. ANA, RA factor, etc. for any immunological problem associated.

5. Factors indicating hypercoagulation, such as protein S, protein C deficiency, anticardiolipin antibodies, hyperhomocysteinemia, etc.

6. 2D echocardiography to rule out source of embolization from heart chambers and valves.

7. Duplex ultrasound scanning of proximal major arteries and aorta as source of embolization.

8. *CT angiography/ DSA:* Typically shows involvement of digital, palmar, plantar arteries with skip areas, normal proximal arteries, and corkscrew collaterals (which are also seen in scleroderma, rheumatoid vasculitis, SLE, antiphospholipid antibody syndrome).

Biopsy is usually not required. But in acute cases with thrombophlebitis, biopsy of short segment of vein will show typical histopathological picture of TAO, which should be diagnostic.

Therapy

Mainstay of treatment is total cessation of smoking or use of tobacco in any form, which has got a lasting benefit. Other treatment modalities are palliative. Even passive smoking may be responsible for continuation of the disease activity. Cessation of smoking leads to decrease in pain intensity, healing of ulcers and decreased rate of amputation. Presence of urinary cotinine indicates that the person has not stopped smoking, which is responsible for the continued worsening of the disease status.

1. Prostaglandin therapy PGI and PGE are available for treatment. It is given in the form of intravenous infusion over 6 hours period daily once and continued for 28 days. In some trials this therapy has led to decrease in pain and

ulcer healing in critical limb ischemia patients. This is to be followed by oral prostaglandin 100-200 microgram twice daily for nearly 8 weeks. Though pain relief is equal in both intravenous and oral therapy, initial IV therapy produces better ulcer healing, but patient needs to remain indoor and the cost of the therapy is high. When other definitive therapy is available prostaglandin therapy is usually deferred.

2. General care of foot and ulcer is essential in all TAO patients due to compromised blood flow.

3. Pentoxifylline (popular brand is Trental 400 mg used thrice daily) has been in use for long time, but the action is no better than placebo in many trials. Hence, it is not being used regularly by vascular specialists.

    Cilostazol is PDE3 inhibitor drug, which has many beneficial actions. It is vasodilator, decreases platelet adhesiveness, reduces lipids and increases blood flow. Given in the dose of 100 mg twice daily over few months produces pain relief, ulcer healing. Initial relief takes few days to weeks. This drug is being commonly used with good clinical benefit.

    Calcium channel blocker like nifedipine and amlodipine are helpful in reducing vasospasm, which is seen in about 40% patients of TAO and should be continued on long-term basis. It is also helpful to treat hypertension, if associated.

    Antiplatelet drugs like aspirin and clopidogrel are advised if proximal major arteries are involved usually in combined atherosclerosis in which case addition of lipid lowering agents is also advised.

4. *Sympathectomy:* This is not usually advised as the benefits are not clearly defined. It may occasionally help in healing of superficial ulcers, but the amputation rate is not altered and the benefit of the procedure is short lasting.

5. *Revascularization:* As in TAO most distal vessels are involved and in late cases fibrotic, thrombotic changes occur, these

subjects are usually not suitable for revascularization. In anatomically suitable cases, where there is some luminal patency and skip lesion, revascularization in the form of either angioplasty or surgical bypass using reversed saphenous vein graft can be done. But cessation of smoking is must for long-term benefit.

6. *Neoangiogenesis:* This therapy is tried in desperate situations where amputation is the only remedy left. Before amputation, this modality is worth trying. Vascular endothelial growth factor VEGF 2 or 4 mg dose is given by intramuscular injections at different sites in affected limb. Second dose is given after 4 weeks' interval. Other methods which can produce neovascularization are omental graft, bone marrow transplant, drilling holes in periosteum like in Ilizarov therapy. Any one of these may be tried in a desperate situation, though the results are unpredictable.

7. Intra-arterial thrombolysis has been tried by some and may be effective before thrombus gets organized. But in fully evolved TAO it is less like to be of benefit.

Summary

Definitive therapy is to stop smoking for sure. In majority cilostazol, aspirin, amlodipine on long-term basis may give some relief. Revascularization can be tried in suitable candidates. Aim of therapy is to avoid amputation. Hence neoangiogenesis, prostaglandins all can be tried to save limb.

Extremity Vascular Trauma

Epidemiology

With increasing population more people are on roads with increasing number of vehicles and consequently causing more number of accidents. Similarly increasing number of conflicts among frustrated citizens causes more number of assaults. Thus due to growing number of assaults and accidents day by day more and more vascular trauma cases are getting admitted to hospitals. Vascular trauma is responsible for approximately 3% of total admissions for injury. People less than 45 years of age form about 80% of the group. Young males are affected more as they are more involved in high-risk activities and mortality rate is seven fold higher in males as compared to females.

Ninety percent of vascular injuries occur in extremities. In World War II most of the arterial injuries were treated by ligation. Hence amputation rate was more than 70%. With development of techniques of vascular reconstruction, amputation rate dropped to less than 10%. But due to associated skeletal, soft tissue and nerve injury, long-term disability may occur in 20-50% patients, which may remain a persistent problem despite all advances.

Etiology

Knowing the mechanism of injury is important for treating vascular surgeon for planning diagnostic and treatment modalities. There are usually two types of vascular injuries:

1. *Penetrating injuries* occur due to knives, gunshot wounds. Iatrogenic causes like vascular access may also produce penetrating though localized injury. In one series of penetrating injuries, 64% were due to gunshot wounds; 24% due to knife wounds and 12% due to shot gun blasts. Thus penetrating injuries were more common.

2. *Blunt injuries* typically occur due to vehicular accidents, falls and assaults, etc. Blunt trauma produces diffuse injury to not only vessels but also to soft tissues, bones, nerves, etc. Fracture of bones or dislocation of joints may injure nearby nerves or vessels. Dislocation of knee and elbow joint is more likely to produce such injury.

Biomechanics of Vascular Trauma

Following blunt trauma tissue injury is produced by local compression or rapid deceleration. In penetrating trauma injury is produced by crushing and separation of tissues along the path of penetrating object. Severity of the injury is proportional to the kinetic energy transferred to the tissues, which is a function of the mass and velocity: $KE = M \times V2/2$. (KE: Kinetic energy; M: Mass; V: Velocity)

In penetrating gunshot wound; alteration in velocity affects transfer of KE more than the mass.

In blunt trauma rapid acceleration or deceleration causes body to move away from object causing cavitation, putting extreme strain on points of anatomical fixation. This causes injury to soft tissues, bones and vessels even away from the site of trauma.

Pathophysiology

Arterial injury may present in one of the following four ways:
1. External bleeding
2. Ischemia
3. Pulsatile hematoma
4. Internal bleeding.

External Bleeding

It is a rare form of presentation occurring usually in extremity vascular trauma due to gunshot injury or crush injury with major tissue loss. Such patients present in state of shock and bleeding may stop temporarily due to hypotension. After resuscitation bleeding may start again.

Ischemia

Most common form of presentation in extremity arterial injury is ischemia occurring due to total occlusion of axial or major artery of the limb. This may occur after penetrating or blunt injury.

Pulsatile Hematoma

It may occur due to partial transaction of major artery with overlying tissue cover which produces pulsatile hematoma.

Internal Bleeding

Hemorrhage may be concealed in chest, abdomen and pelvis, in soft tissues of gluteal region or thigh. In facial injuries blood may be swallowed and may remain unnoticed. On investigations such concealed bleeding may be suspected and further evaluated.

Types or Patterns of Vascular Injury

Most common type is arterial laceration with complete or incomplete transaction. Incomplete transaction leads to hemorrhage which may be severe and continuous. In complete transaction ends of the injured artery get thrombosed and retract, thus stopping bleeding. There may be intimal injury which leads to delayed thrombosis. Pseudoaneurysm may form with bleeding in surrounding tissue which gets localized. Arteriovenous fistula may form if artery and vein which are closely related, are injured.

Clinical Features

Signs of arterial injury are divided in two major categories.
1. Hard signs are as follows:
    •   Absence of distal pulsations
    •   Active external bleeding
    •   Signs of ischemia
    •   Pulsatile hematoma
    •   Bruit/thrill over or near the artery.
2. Soft signs are as follows:
    •   Diminished distal pulsations
    •   Injury in the proximity of major artery
    •   Neurological deficit
    •   Hypotension or shock.

Clinical examination should include inspection, palpation and auscultation to identify signs of acute ischemia.

Arteriovenous fistula, pseudoaneurysm should be suspected following a penetrating injury in the presence of pulsatile hematoma accompanied by a bruit or thrill.

In patients with soft signs, ankle brachial index (ABI) of 0.9 or less should prompt further work up.

Bony injury, other injuries like thoracic, abdominal injuries should be suspected in relevant cases, which may take priority in treatment.

Diagnostic Evaluation

On admission blood sample should be withdrawn for Hb, CBC, platelet count, KFT, electrolytes, blood group and BSL. Adequate amount of blood should be cross matched. Seropositivity and Australia antigen are routinely tested these days as before any operation.

X-ray of the extremity for long bone fracture should be taken. Because certain fractures like the ones around knee and elbow have high incidence of neurovascular injury (Figs 5.1 and 5.2).

Patients with extremity vascular injury have varied clinical presentation. Patients who present with hard signs of arterial injury like pulsatile external bleeding, enlarging hematoma, absent distal pulses, arterial ischemia need immediate arterial exploration without further diagnostic evaluation. Intraoperative angiography is preferred in such cases.

Most arterial injuries are however clinically not evident and need further diagnostic evaluation.

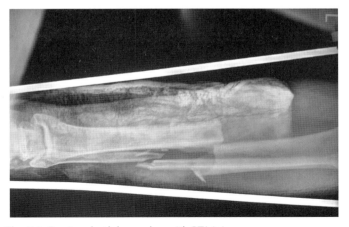

Fig. 5.1: Fracture both bones leg with PTA injury

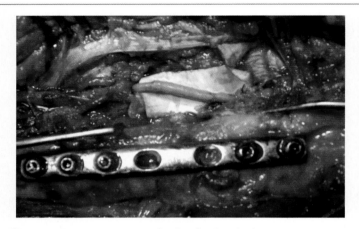

Fig. 5.2: PTA interposition graft. Tibia fixed with plate

Duplex ultrasound with color Doppler imaging of the injured extremity is a valuable investigation. It is easily available in many centers, it is easy to perform, can be repeated and complications associated with arteriography are avoided. It is a good screening technique, which is sufficient in many cases for assessment. It can even be performed bedside, in case patient cannot be shifted due to comorbidity.

However, it cannot be performed in patients with plasters, splints, external fixators, with large tissue and skin loss causing raw area. Expertise is required to give authentic and reliable report which should help the vascular surgeon in planning exploration.

Angiography: It is advised in patients who are clinically, hemo-dynamically stable, KFT is satisfactory and depending on soft signs exploration is likely to be required. It may identify patients who may be benefitted by endovascular intervention rather than exploration.

The ABI is a simple reliable method of assessing arterial injury. The ABI of 0.9 or less indicates ischemia. However it does not localize the site of injury, but it is definitely more sensitive than only digital palpation of peripheral arteries. It is a simple reproducible method of screening arterial injury.

CT scan is usually not advised for extremity vascular injury.

Management

Nonoperative Management

Patients with soft signs or minimal nonocclusive arterial injury (on angiographic evaluation), clinically asymptomatic patients may be observed. But indication of surgery may develop anytime during observation period. Then treatment must be accordingly modified. Some authors think aggressively even to explore all these patients, but majority are in favor of conservative treatment. About 87% of such patients have been found to have good healing of arterial injury or good resolution of thrombus over 1-12 weeks period. Hence there is a definite place for nonoperative management of such patients.

Patients with partial thrombosis, associated venous injury are benefitted with low molecular weight heparin/anticoagulant. If artificial graft is interposed, postoperative LMWH and antiplatelet agents form mainstay of medical treatment, if there is no contraindication.

Endovascular Management

Transcatheter embolization of coils or balloons can be tried in selected situations like post-traumatic arteriovenous fistula (AVF), low flow false aneurysms and to occlude peripheral non-accessible arteries to arrest bleeding from artery occlusion of which would not cause ischemia and gangrene. Coils are made from stainless steel and tufted with wool or Dacron. These coils are useful to occlude peripheral bleeding artery and AVF, when introduced through 5F or 7F size catheter. After deployment coils expand and occlude the desired site. Dacron or wool tuft promotes thrombosis. If blood flow persists after 5 minutes, second coil is deployed. In case of AVF coil is lodged on venous side keeping the supplying artery patent. The diameter of the coil should match that of vessel embolized to avoid distal migration. Barium impregnated silicone like beads were also used successfully in trauma patients.

Recently by putting artificial graft with stent by endovascular technique, false aneurysm, AVF and arterial injury have been repaired (Fig. 5.3). It is a promising technique in selected patients, especially when surgical intervention could be of high risk. Experience is accumulating in favor of this modality and it may become procedure of choice in future when the facility and expertise are made available for stent graft deployment on

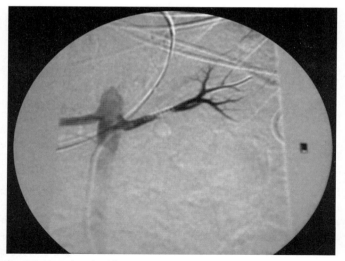

Fig. 5.3: Vascular stent in trauma

regular basis, at even peripheral centers and at affordable cost to the majority.

Operative Treatment

Regional anesthesia is preferred for majority, unless the patient is unstable or noncooperative. The complete extremity is cleaned and draped and the opposite limb is prepared for autogenous great saphenous vein if required for grafting. If the vessel is not lying exposed due to injury, proximal and distal ends of the artery are exposed and controlled. Injection heparin 1 mg per kg of body weight is given intravenously as a bolus to prevent thrombus formation or propagation if already formed. Standard contraindications must be verified before giving heparin like major bleed or intracranial bleed. Both arterial ends are debrided and freshened till normal intima is seen and then the ends are secured by bulldog vascular clamps. If the arterial ends are not seen or controlled easily, under fluoroscopic guidance percutaneously passed balloon catheter can be used to occlude the bleeding end or preoperatively Fogarty balloon catheter is passed and balloon inflated to control bleeding. After freshening arterial ends, Fogarty catheter of appropriate size is passed ante grade and retrograde to clear thrombi and to have good flow. Both ends are mobilized to reach each other, if required after sacrificing few minor branches. Then end to end anastomosis is done using 5-0 or 6-0 polypropylene suture in a continuous manner. For smaller artery even 7-0 suture may be required. The anastomosis should be free from tension, leak and kink. In case the artery is partially transected, edges are freshened and rent repaired with polypropylene suture. If a gap of more than 2 cm results after debridement of injured arterial ends, direct anastomosis is not possible and interposition graft using reversed great saphenous vein from the opposite normal limb should ideally be used (Figs 5.4 to 5.6). If the ipsilateral leg is not injured, then RSVG from even the same side may be used.

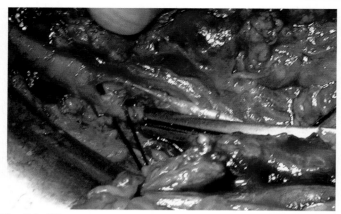

Fig. 5.4: CFA tear

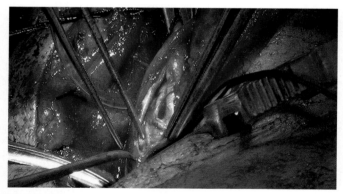

Fig. 5.5: SFA tear

For above knee bypass polytetrafluoroethylene (PTFE) of 6 or 8 mm size may be used with good long-term patency, but for below knee bypass RSVG is the best conduit.

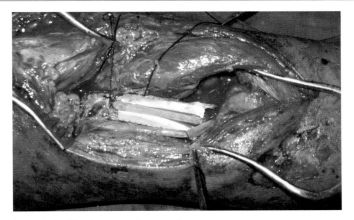

Fig. 5.6: Popliteal interposition graft

If management of associated injuries like soft tissue, fractured long bones, repair of nerves, etc. is anticipated, revascularization may be delayed considerably increasing ischemia time. To tide over this problem, temporary intra-arterial shunt should be used to maintain arterial flow till the final repair.

Extra-anatomical graft is used in patients having associated extensive soft tissue injury or sepsis.

Vein injury if partial, can be repaired by lateral venorrhaphy. In case transaction, both ends must be securely ligated. Anastomosis using interposition graft has not been found to be useful in anyway. The same may get thrombosed.

In case the patient is very unstable due major associated injuries or due to major bleed and cannot withstand major surgical intervention lasting for long time, ligation of bleeding artery and veins is useful to control bleed to save life, though not the limb. Associated skeletal injury is taken care of by orthopedic surgeon and nerve repair and soft tissue cover if required is accomplished by plastic surgeon. Soft tissue cover is mandatory for arterial revascularization, nerve repair and bone implants. Thus, it is a team approach that is required to salvage the limb and life.

In case of combined arterial and venous injury or delayed ischemia, fracture of long bones, preoperative compartment syndrome, fasciotomy to release all the compartments must be done. In case of dilemma of doing or not doing, it must be done.

Sometimes, the patient presents with severely damaged, crushed extremity, where Mangled Extremity Severity Score (MESS) is high. There is extensive loss of soft tissue, bones are fractured, and there is gross wound contamination and extensive nerve injury, amputation remains the best option to save life and to avoid morbidity. Amputation is also likely to be required for occluded bypass graft, combined above knee and below knee injury, a tense compartment with arterial transaction and compound fractures. In such cases amputation improves general condition quickly so that further measures can be adapted.

Thoracic Outlet Syndrome

This is a symptom complex occurring in upper extremity due to compression of neurovascular structures in thoracic outlet. Compressed structures are brachial plexus, subclavian artery and vein. Compressing structures are cervical rib, first rib, fibromuscular elements, etc. The areas affected are scalene triangle and costoclavicular space.

Three types of thoracic outlet syndromes (TOS) are recognized as follows:

1. Neurogenic TOS
2. Arterial TOS
3. Venous TOS.

Symptoms produced by vascular TOS are typical and clinical diagnosis is easy, while neurogenic TOS has vague symptoms and diagnosis is difficult and elusive. Overall vascular signs are more while neurogenic symptoms are more.

Anatomy (Fig. 6.1)

1. Scalene triangle
2. Costoclavicular space.

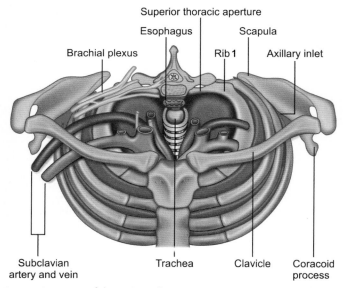

Fig. 6.1: Anatomy of thoracic outlet

Etiology

Arterial TOS

It forms nearly 1% of all TOS cases. It is usually caused by the complete cervical rib or rudimentary first rib. About 88% of these patients have bony abnormality, which is rare in asymptomatic individuals. Complete cervical rib articulates with the superior surface of 1st rib lateral to the insertion of scalenus anticus muscle. Across this site subclavian artery (SCA) courses and gets stretched, which produces intimal injury. The later can throw emboli in distal arterial circulation. Later on aneurysm may form. Long transverse process of C7 cervical vertebra, partial cervical rib may also produce SCA compression. Whatever is the cause, repetitive use of arm and neck muscles (e.g. sports, some professions like painters, etc.) appears to be important precipitating cause for producing symptoms.

Venous TOS

It forms nearly 5% of all TOS cases. Thrombosis of subclavian-axillary vein occurs due to compression of subclavian vein (SCV) at costoclavicular space, which is the medial most part of the thoracic outlet. Compression leads to stasis, intimal injury and thrombosis. Repetitive arm and shoulder actions predispose to thrombosis. Costoclavicular ligament and hypertrophied subclavius muscle may cause compression of SCV in some patients.

Neurogenic TOS

It is the most common type of TOS, which occurs because of compression of five components of brachial plexus in scalene triangle. Surprisingly normal anatomy of scalene triangle is found in many such individuals despite clinical symptoms suggestive of neurogenic TOS. Hyperabduction of arm and hyperextension of neck, repetitively, enhance the injury to brachial plexus due to repeated compression. The associated abnormalities, if present, only help to increase the likelihood of injury. This injury causes chronic inflammation of scalenus anticus muscle, which leads to spasm, then fibrosis with contracture. Hence, it becomes stiff causing irritation of nerve roots and producing symptoms. But it must be clearly stated that the exact pathophysiology of neurogenic TOS is not clearly understood.

Various abnormalities associated with TOS are as listed below:

A. *Bony abnormalities:*
   i. *Congenital:* Cervical rib, long C7 transverse process, 1st rib abnormalities
   ii. *Acquired:* Fracture of 1st rib, clavicle with callus, tumor, and exostosis

B. *Soft tissue abnormalities:*
   i. *Congenital:* Abnormal insertions/hypertrophy of scalenus anticus and medius, abnormal ligaments and fascial bands, etc. scalenus minimus muscle.
   ii. *Acquired:* Neck trauma, previous surgery with fibrosis, scalenus muscle trauma, reattachment of scalenus insertion, soft tissue tumor, etc.

C. *Brachial plexus*:
   i. Congenital defects, pre-and-postfixed brachial plexus
   ii. Acquired like schwannoma, surgery on brachial plexus, etc.

D. Postural defects can occur due to various professions, sagging of shoulders, heavy breasts, etc.

Clinical Features

Neurogenic TOS

This occurs in patient age group of 20-40 years and more than 75% are females. Individuals involved in activities requiring elevation of arms or excessive neck movements are prone to develop symptoms.

1. *Pain:* Usually occurs anywhere from hand to shoulder without localization. It may be associated with numbness, weakness, paresthesia which may be localized depending on which part of the brachial plexus is compressed. Upper trunk involvement produces symptoms along the distribution of radial and musculocutaneous nerves and lower trunk involvement along the ulnar and median

nerves. Symptoms are mild and intermittent in many, but fear of pain may produce muscular wasting or atrophy due to avoidance of activity. This may occur in extreme cases.

2. *Headache:* Usually occurs in occipital area and is due to spasm and referred pain from traphezius and paraspinal muscles. However, the headache due to migraine and neurogenic TOS may coexist adding difficulty for differentiation.

3. *Vascular symptoms:* Patients may initially present with symptoms suggestive of secondary Raynaud's syndrome like discoloration and coldness of hand and fingers due to vasospasm. There could be hypersensitivity to touch and even causalgia. Arterial emboli lodged in distal digital arteries produce pain in fingertips and blue discoloration. Thrombotic occlusion of artery produces ulceration and gangrene.

In venous TOS males predominate with 2:1 proportion, average age is 31 years. Dominant arm is involved in more than 75% cases and 75% give history of strenuous/repetitive activity involving that arm before the onset of symptoms.

Physical Examination

Neurogenic TOS

The clinical examination in neurogenic TOS carries a great importance as the diagnosis is usually elusive and examination findings and assessment are really helpful. Diagnosis is usually by exclusion. Ulnar nerve entrapment at elbow and median nerve compression at wrist in carpal tunnel syndrome should be ruled out. Localized tenderness beyond scalene triangle like in neck, traphezius muscle, shoulder, etc. must be noted which suggests other possibilities.

Supraclavicular tenderness on specific trigger points in scalene triangle may produce typical symptoms. Spasm of scalenus anticus may be appreciated after tapping on this point which is suggestive of TOS.

Roos' EAST (Elevated Arm Stress Test): It is performed with arm elevated above head and fist is opened and closed repeatedly. Normal person can perform this action for several minutes, while in neurogenic TOS the subject experiences fatigue, pain and numbness in arm and digits within 30-50 seconds.

Arterial TOS

There may be palpable cervical rib in posterior triangle felt as bony mass along with pulsatile supraclavicular lesion suggestive of subclavian artery aneurysm. Bruit may be heard over the aneurysm. Signs of ischemia of digits may be present like blue discoloration of tips, ulceration, and cold temperature. Peripheral pulsations may be absent. Some positional maneuvers which increase the compression of SCA are as follows:

a. *Adson's test:* Patient is made to sit erect with arms hanging by the side and is asked to inspire deeply, hyperextend the neck and turn to opposite side. If radial pulse disappears, the test is said to be positive, which is due to compression of SCA by cervical rib and scalenus anticus muscle. But it must be noted that the test may be positive in 15-55% of normal individuals.

b. *Costoclavicular compression or military position:* Here shoulders are depressed and pulled backwards which causes compression of SCA in costoclavicular space between 1st rib and clavicle. If radial pulse disappears the test is positive.

c. Hyperabduction test is carried out with hyperabduction of shoulder during which axillary artery is compressed by pectoralis minor.

It must be clearly understood that the positional tests do not have diagnostic reliability.

Venous TOS

Majority of the patients are young, involved extremity is dominant extremity and after precipitating event, i.e. excessive use of arm, patient usually presents within 24 hours with acute swelling of upper limb with cyanosis and pain. Without features of deep vein thrombosis diagnosis of venous compression clinically may not be possible.

Diagnostic Evaluation

In neurogenic TOS most tests are done to exclude other conditions to help diagnosis by exclusion. The importance of thorough clinical examination cannot be overemphasized.

  i. Plain X-ray neck shows rudimentary or complete cervical rib, abnormalities of 1st rib, long transverse process of C7 cervical vertebra and callus/fracture or any other abnormality of clavicle. In addition degenerative changes in cervical spine can be diagnosed. Thus, a good quality X-ray can help in diagnosis of osseous abnormalities.

 ii. *Imaging modality like MRI, CT scan:* These are helpful to diagnose degenerative cervical spine disease, intracranial disease, shoulder abnormalities, etc. MRI may diagnose hypertrophied scalenus anticus muscle, prominent ligaments and fibrous bands in scalene triangle and also structural abnormalities in brachial plexus.

iii. *Nerve conduction velocity (NCV) and electromyography (EMG):* Results of NCV, EMG are usually normal in neurogenic TOS as nerve roots are compressed quite proximally and intermittently. Hence permanent damage may not occur early in course of disease. However positive test results indicate advanced disease and poor outcome of treatment.

iv. *Scalene muscle block:* Injecting local anesthetic in scalenus anticus muscle belly produces relief of muscle spasm and consequently the symptoms in arm and hand. The positive test indicates that the surgery is going to be of help in such patient. This test is useful if diagnosis is equivocal. But if the local anesthesia also affects brachial plexus, the test result is not reliable.

v. *Duplex ultrasound (DUS):* In normal posture and with arm hyper- extended can demonstrate SCA compression. Intimal irregularity, aneurysm, subclavian vein thrombosis all can be reliably demonstrated by DUS.

vi. *Angiography:* This is rarely required for diagnosis (Figs 6.2A and B). If intervention is planned, contrast angiography is essential. It can demonstrate compression of SCA in a particular posture. Also intimal irregularity, aneurysm, occlusion and distal reformation or run off, which are essential for planning intervention, are all visualized on angiography. Similarly contrast venography can demonstrate SCV compression in costoclavicular space before actual thrombosis occurs.

Differential Diagnosis

- Cervical disk lesion with nerve root compression
- Soft tissue strain in neck region due to excessive physical exertion or sprain
- Shoulder arthritis or tendon lesions
- Spinal cord tumor, multiple sclerosis
- Fibromyalgia of traphezius, rhomboid muscle, etc.
- Raynaud's syndrome, sympathetic disease, etc.

Management

Conservative Management

Initial treatment in all neurogenic TOS is conservative. The same is also required to be continued after operation for few weeks. Experienced physiotherapist is mandatory for success of conservative treatment, otherwise symptoms may worsen.

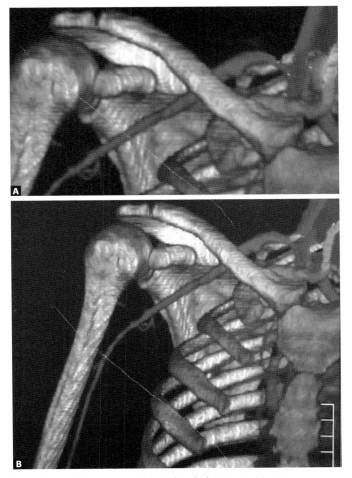

Figs 6.2A and B: Thoracic outlet with subclavian angiogram

It consists of pain relieving therapy to supraclavicular area and therapy to improve muscle strength of neck and upper extremity. Relaxation of the neck muscles is also to be taught. Therapy is continued minimum for 6 weeks and result is analyzed. If satisfactory relief is obtained the same is continued further. If not, patient is reassessed. Therapy can be combined with hydrotherapy, massage, etc. Posture correction is taught to avoid sagging of shoulders. Training of abdominal breathing is given to avoid excessive strain on neck muscles. Heavy breasts are properly supported.

In conservative treatment drugs used are analgesics, antidepressants and muscle relaxants, which are useful in chronic cases.

If a particular occupation is responsible for symptoms, change of job or profession is helpful.

Many patients get relief with conservative treatment as above.

Surgical Management

It is indicated if conservative management fails after adequate trial for about 3 months and if the neurological symptoms worsen to the extent of causing interference in daily routine activities.

Aims of treatment are:
  i. To relieve all factors causing neurovascular compression.
 ii. Restore arterial continuity.
iii. To achieve SCV patency.

Transaxillary Approach

Roos in 1966 devised this approach for 1st rib resection. It is done by high transverse incision in axilla. As the arm is abducted, nerves and vessels are retracted away from the 1st rib. Anterior scalene muscle is divided close to insertion on scalene tubercle saving phrenic nerve. Scalenus medius is pushed off. Nerve root of T1 is identified and protected and first rib is resected.

Advantages: It is a cosmetic incision. Soft tissue compression and that due to 1st rib is removed. Adequate decompression of the costoclavicular space is achieved.

Disadvantages: This needs very strong retraction of arm and limited exposure of thoracic outlet is obtained. Radical scalenotomy is not possible. Posterior segment of 1st rib and cervical rib are difficult to remove. Long thoracic nerve may be damaged. Vascular injury cannot be taken care of, which may, sometimes, become life-threatening.

Hence, these days, it is not a preferred approach.

Supraclavicular Approach

This approach gives opportunity for radical decompression of thoracic outlet of any etiology.

Radical scalenotomy is possible. All osseous compression due to cervical rib, first rib, and medial end of clavicle can be taken care of. All musculotendinous compressing bands can be removed from the scalene triangle to free brachial plexus. Interventions on SCA and SCV are possible through the same approach. Cervical sympathectomy if required for vasospastic symptoms can be easily carried out.

Some people have advised combined supraclavicular and axillary approach to achieve good decompression of upper and lower trunks. By supraclavicular approach scalenotomy, neurolysis and excision of osseous compression are taken care of and by axillary approach 1st rib is excised and lower trunk is freed better. In a deserving case, the combined approach may be utilized.

Management of Arterial TOS

By supraclavicular approach compressing elements like cervical rib usually and sometimes 1st rib are excised after dissecting and protecting SCA. Sometimes medial claviculectomy may be required. Anterior scalene muscle is excised from insertion. Scalenus medius is also similarly divided. Arterial lesions can be dealt in following ways:

i. Arteriotomy is done. If only plaque is found, intima should be excised to prevent embolization.

ii. If artery is thrombosed with soft thrombus and intima is normal, embolectomy with Fogarty balloon catheter is adequate. Intra-arterial thrombolysis with urokinase, if added, improves result. There should be good back flow at the end of the procedure. If the balloon catheter is not negotiated easily up to wrist, separate arteriotomy at brachial bifurcation is required.

iii. Poststenotic fusiform dilatation can be reduced by linear arteriotomy and closure to narrow the lumen at affected site.

iv. Aneurysm requires resection and interposition of reversed great saphenous vein from thigh or artificial graft of 6-8 mm diameter (PTFE).

v. In chronic occlusions and distally good run off in arm/ forearm arteries, bypass using reversed great saphenous vein should be carried with patent distal artery as assessed on angiography. If proximal SCA segment is short, common carotid artery can be used as inflow artery and bypass done to distal SCA or axillary artery.

Management of Venous TOS

Patient is usually asymptomatic with intermittent SCV compression. Young male patient presents with acute swelling, pain, cyanosis of dominant upper extremity occurring after repetitive activity. The diagnosis of subclavian vein thrombosis is clinically evident. Catheter directed thrombolysis with urokinase is started with a bolus of 2.5 lac units, 4000 units in next 1 hour followed by 1000 units per hour for next 24 hours. Clot lysis is assessed. If it is incomplete, thrombolysis is continued further or transluminal balloon venoplasty can be done. Once the patient is stabilized, compressing 1st rib or medial clavicular end must be excised for lasting result. Otherwise 75% patients have residual venous hypertension and symptoms.

In chronic SCV thrombosis by planned supraclavicular approach 1st rib or medial end of clavicle is removed. In the same sitting SCV thrombectomy is done and venotomy closed. Long term results are good with this procedure.

In both acute and chronic cases anticoagulation is continued for 3-6 months.

Complications of Surgery

1. *Nerve injury:* Injury to brachial plexus is likely due to strong retraction and stretching or direct injury, which is more likely with transaxillary approach. Recovery occurs within next 3 months in majority.

2. Lymphatic injury leading to leakage may occur for some time.

3. Recurrence of symptoms due to either incomplete resection of osseous compression or reattachment of scalenus anticus is also likely.

Raynaud's Syndrome

Historical Background

In 1882, Maurice Raynaud, a French physician submitted a thesis which contained the description of the entity affecting upper extremity causing episodes of pallor of fingertips followed by cyanosis and then rubor. He described that the changes occurred due to sympathetic over activity and were precipitated by exposure to cold or emotional stress. This disease entity was later named after him as "Raynaud`s Disease."

In 1901, Hutchinson postulated that there could be multiple causes responsible for this clinical picture apart from just exposure to cold and emotional stress.

Terminology and Definition

Raynaud`s syndrome (RS) is defined as episodic pallor or cyanosis of fingers due to vasoconstriction of small arteries or arterioles in the fingers occurring in response to exposure to cold or emotional stress.

Initially two terminologies were used:
1. *Raynaud's disease:* Refers to primary vasospastic disorder where no identifiable cause is found.
2. *Raynaud's phenomenon:* Here, vasospasm is secondary to underlying cause or condition.

In actual clinical practice, these two terms were commonly interchanged. Hence to avoid the confusion, the nomenclature 'Raynaud's syndrome' has been suggested.

Now primary RS indicates clinical syndrome where vasospasm is primary and secondary RS includes patients who have underlying cause, e.g. TAO, atherosclerosis, etc.

Prevalence of Raynaud's Syndrome

It is difficult to give accurate incidence of RS in general population because it could be a normal phenomenon in many and many with mild symptoms may not report to the hospital as the episode is short-lasting and self-limiting. In various studies incidence of 3.5 to 4.5% has been found in general population. In cooler regions, there is a higher prevalence, could be up to 10%. It commonly affects females of younger age groups. But recent survey indicates the male to female ratio of 1:1.6. Most commonly fingers are involved but both fingers and toes are affected in up to one-third cases. Coronary and cerebral circulation may also be affected by vasospasm causing Prinzmetal's angina and migraine headaches respectively.

Pathophysiology

Primary Raynaud's Syndrome

Exact cause of episodic vasospasm is not clearly understood. Whether there is a local factor responsible or the thermoregulatory mechanism is exaggerated in response to exposure to cold remains uncertain. Local, humoral, and nervous mechanisms could be responsible for vasoconstriction.

In response to stimulation sympathetic nerve endings secrete norepinephrine, this acts on the postjunctional alpha-2 receptors which are located in vascular smooth muscle cells. This initiates vasoconstriction. This normal response is probably exaggerated by exposure to cold producing intense vasoconstriction.

There may be underlying endothelial dysfunction causing decreased release of nitric oxide which is a potent vasodilator and increased release of endothelin-1 which is a vasoconstrictor. Imbalance between these two factors can cause enhanced vasoconstriction.

Platelets may also be involved in producing vasospasm. Activated platelets release thromboxane A_2 and serotonin both of which may enhance vasospasm.

These mechanisms decrease intraluminal distending pressure and thereby decrease critical closing pressure (pressure at which artery is occluded due to spasm), thus producing spasm due to this imbalance. When endothelial derived contracting factor (EDCF) exceeds endothelial derived relaxing factor (EDRF) vasospasm occurs. After vasospasm occurs due to exposure to cold, emotional stress or smoking, fingertips become pale. Later on due to further desaturation of stagnated blood in pulp space of fingers cyanosis occurs (Fig. 7.1). After sometime cold induced vasodilatation occurs and blood starts flowing producing red color or rubor. Thus typical tricolor changes occur in sequence. However, all the color changes may not occur in every patient. Episode may last for a few minutes and is usually over by 20 minutes.

Coffman has summarized criteria for primary RS as follows:

1. Typical episode precipitated by cold exposure, emotional stress
2. Bilateral affection of upper limbs
3. Absence of gangrene
4. Duration of symptoms minimum 2 years
5. Absence of any identifiable cause.

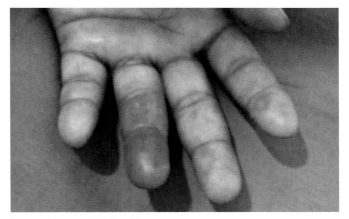

Fig. 7.1: Vasculitis of ring finger

Secondary Raynaud's Syndrome

Various causes are associated with secondary RS. They are as follows:

1. Arterial occlusive diseases like atherosclerosis, TAO, thoracic outlet syndrome, giant cell arteritis and embolization
2. Connective tissue disorders (CTD) like scleroderma, CREST syndrome, SLE, rheumatoid arthritis, dermatomyositis, etc.
3. Malignancy like multiple myeloma, adenocarcinoma, leukemia, etc.
4. Hematological disorders like cold agglutinins, cryoglobulinemia, thrombocytosis, polycythemia rubra, etc.
5. Secondary to drugs like beta adrenergic blockers, ergot, cocaine, vasopressors, anticancer drugs, etc.
6. Infection like hepatitis B and C, parvovirus, etc.

Scleroderma is the most common CTD causing fibrosis of skin, internal organs and of small vessels. Joints are affected.

Ulcers occur over joints and fingertips which are slow to heal which produce significant pain. Rheumatoid arthritis may also cause small vessel fibrosis. TAO may produce vasospasm initially in 30-40% individuals. Atherosclerosis produces chronic symptoms when occlusive, otherwise intermittent symptoms may occur due to peripheral emboli. Later picture may also be produced by arterial TOS. Hence, individual case needs to be evaluated based on its clinical presentation.

Clinical Features

Subject is usually young female who complains of pallor of fingertips on exposure to cold or emotional stress which becomes blue and then red within few minutes. There is usually numbness, paresthesia but no pain or ulcer and the attack subsides leaving no tissue damage. Recurrent episodes may occur. In scleroderma, the features are as described above. History of smoking in a male patient presenting with fingertip gangrene points to TAO as the possible cause. Palpable cervical rib with subclavian artery aneurysm points towards arterial TOS as the cause for arterial emboli. In older individuals with features of RS having evidence occlusion of lower limb pulsations atherosclerosis as the probable cause must be thought. Digital ulcers, joint deformity, shiny tight skin is suggestive of scleroderma. Hence, all these findings must be looked for during examination.

Noninvasive Diagnostic Studies

Many noninvasive tests have been described for the diagnosis of RS, but majority do not give conclusive result, e.g. measurement of finger systolic pressure or segmental pressure, fingertip thermography, etc. Some of the tests of diagnostic importance are as follows:

Cold Recovery Time

Using temperature probe baseline digital temperature is recorded at the end of finger pulp. Then hands are immersed in cold water at 4°C for 20 seconds. Then hands are dried and pulp temperature is again recorded. Length of time taken at room temperature to return to baseline temperature is recorded. In normal individuals, this rewarming takes nearly 10 minutes. In patients with RS, it takes longer sometimes up to 30 minutes.

This test cannot differentiate between primary and secondary RS and some have questioned the reliability of this test.

Laser Doppler Flux

Here, instead of temperature probe Laser Doppler probe is used to measure microvascular skin perfusion to fingers. Low powered Helium Neon light emitted by the probe is scattered by moving red blood cells. Frequency shift caused by scattered light is detected by the probe and proportional output signal is produced. Laser Doppler flux is decreased during cooling and increased during rewarming, which is to be compared with normal control.

Laser Doppler after Warming

Most patients with RS present with cold hands. Hence fingers are warmed up to 37°C in a box. Laser Doppler baseline flow and that after rewarming are recorded and compared. Increase in flow is observed 4-5 times in fingers having baseline vasoconstriction. Failure to obtain increase in blood flow after rewarming indicates fixed obstruction and points towards secondary RS.

Imaging Modalities

Duplex ultrasound is helpful in imaging digital arteries and completeness of palmar arch can be assessed specially during Allen's test.

Magnetic resonance angiography is another useful modality, which gives good pictures of digital arteries but resolution is inferior to that of contrast angiography.

Invasive Studies

Contrast angiography is a gold standard but is rarely performed only for diagnostic purpose. It is advised in severe form of RS where interventions like thrombolysis, angioplasty or surgery are anticipated. This can give idea about atheroemboli, arterial emboli for example from aneurysm of subclavian artery, cork-screw collaterals in TAO, vasculitis, etc.

Management

This can be considered under three heads:
- Preventive treatment
- Drug therapy
- Interventions.

Preventive Treatment

Exposure to cold being the commonest factor, it must be avoided by using warm garments. Total body warming should be observed during cold season. Emotional stress should be avoided by self-restrain or by drugs. Smoking or nicotine in any form, ergotamine (for migraine), beta blockers (for hypertension), abused drugs (like cocaine, amphetamine) all of them produce vasoconstriction and hence must be avoided at all costs. Arm rotation sometimes is helpful to avoid attack of vasospasm. These preventive measures are sufficient to avert the episode in majority of the cases.

Drug Therapy

They are reserved for patients having significant symptoms despite preventive measures observed for adequate time.

Calcium channel blockers are the most preferred drugs. Nifedipine sustained preparation 20-30 mg twice daily is usually advised. Side effects like flushing, edema, headache, and tachycardia may force 15% patients to stop therapy. Long-acting preparation like amlodipine 5-10 mg daily also produces good relief. Diltiazem 30-90 mg daily is less potent but has fewer side effects. Secondary RS patients may not have adequate relief. Therapy with calcium channel blockers may be required for approximately 1 year.

Alpha-1 adrenergic blockers are preferred if subject is intolerant to calcium channel blockers. Selective alpha blocker like prazosin can be used in the dose of 1-5 mg 2-3 times daily. Orthostatic hypotension is the common side effect. Hence, lower dose and bed time administration should be preferred. Dorazocin 1-8 mg daily is a long-acting drug.

Recently ACE inhibitor, losartan have also been found to be effective. Fluoxetine 20 mg daily has been shown to produce good relief.

Prostaglandin E, Prostaglandin I_2 infusion has been found to be beneficial in patients with digital ulceration and pain. These are potent vasodilators and inhibitor of platelet aggregation. But the therapy is costly and needs to be continued for a long time.

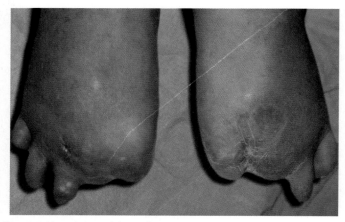

Fig. 7.2: Vasculitis with loss of toes

Interventions

Surgery

Cervicothoracic sympathectomy has been performed in patients with recurrent symptoms and ulceration. Initial benefit may last for about 6 months and then the symptoms recur. As the sympathectomy is beneficial only in vasospastic RS where drugs are equally effective, this procedure is not carried out routinely these days. As this procedure can be carried out thoracoscopically presently with minimum morbidity, it can be carried out in unresponsive patients for short-term relief.

Local debridement is carried out if there is tissue necrosis. Digital amputation may be required in 10-20% patients. Amputation should be avoided as the stump may take a long time for healing. However, local care of the wound is important as in any other case with infection (Fig. 7.2).

Arterial Aneurysms

History

The history of aneurysms dates back to ancient times wherein there is description of pulsatile swellings of the body in *Charaka Samhita*. First documented description of abdominal aortic aneurysm in the literature is in 16th century by Vesalius. Rudolph Matas in 1923 successfully ligated aorta in patient of abdominal aortic aneurysm (AAA). Rea in 1948 made use of cellophane to wrap around neck and anterolateral surface of AAA in order to induce fibrosis and limit expansion. Using this technique, Nissen in 1949 treated AAA of great scientist Albert Einstein. He survived for 6 years after this before he succumbed to ruptured AAA. In 1951, Charles Dubost from Paris, France was the first person to replace AAA using freeze dried homograft. Presently endoaneurysmorrhaphy using a prosthetic graft as originally popularized by Creech, Michael DeBakey and Stanley Crawford, is the commonest procedure for repair of AAA. First successful repair of ruptured AAA was done by Denton Cooley and DeBakey in 1954. Juan Parodi in 1991 performed the first successful endovascular graft repair of AAA.

Definition

Aneurysm is defined as a focal dilatation of an artery greater than 1.5 times its normal diameter (nonaneurysmal segment).

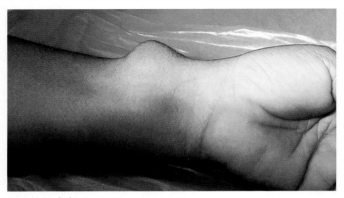

Fig. 8.1: Radial artery aneurysm

Aneurysms can occur anywhere in the body, but the most common locations are abdominal and thoracic aorta, iliac, femoral, popliteal and cerebral arteries (Figs 8.1 to 8.7).

Classification of Aneurysms

Aneurysms are classified based on their shape, wall constituents and etiology.

- Based on shape:
    - *Fusiform:* It is a spindle-shaped; diffuse dilatation of the vessel which is the most common type.
    - *Saccular:* Where one wall of the vessel is dilated producing eccentric aneurysm.
- Wall constituents:
    - *True aneurysm:* It contains all the elements of the arterial wall.
    - *False or pseudoaneurysm:* It contains partly the wall constituents and partly outside/surrounding tissue. Blood leaking from arterial puncture or from vascular anastomosis forms pseudoaneurysm.

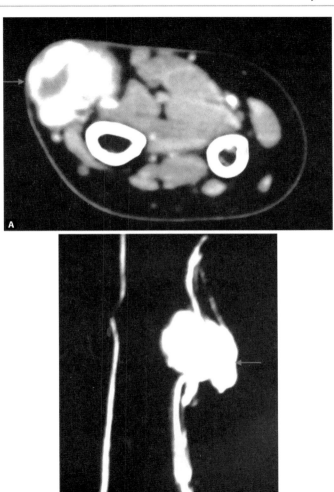

Figs 8.2A and B: Radial artery aneurysm—CT angiogram

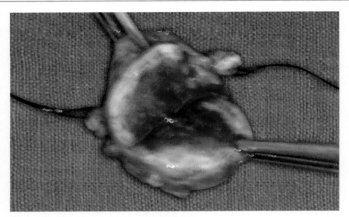

Fig. 8.3: Radial artery aneurysm excised

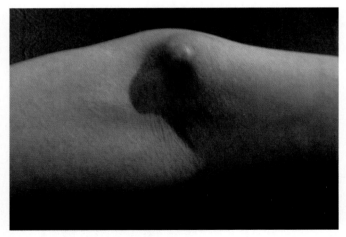

Fig. 8.4: Brachial artery aneurysm

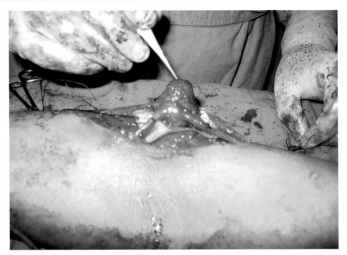

Fig. 8.5: Brachial artery aneurysm—Exposed

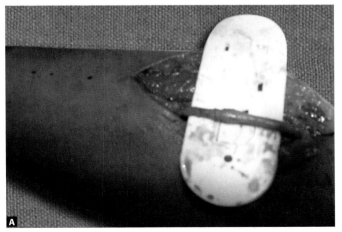

Fig. 8.6A

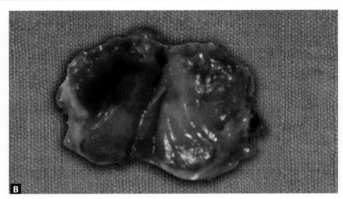

Fig. 8.6B
Figs 8.6A and B: Brachial artery aneurysm—excised and grafted

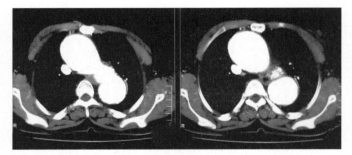

Fig. 8.7: CT angiogram of thoracic aneurysm

- Based on etiology:
  - *Degenerative:* Most common is atherosclerotic aneurysm of abdominal aorta.
  - *Dissecting aneurysm:* Here elements of the vessel wall disrupt and due to weakness thus produced the vessel wall dilates gradually. The blood then flows through the layers producing dissection, which is a mechanism in thoracic aorta.

- *Mycotic aneurysm:* Infection may occur from inside the lumen of the vessel due to infective embolus or from outside infective focus eroding into vessel wall, which produce weakness of vessel wall and produces aneurysm, which is challenging to repair. It is infective aneurysm and the term 'Mycotic' is misnomer.
- *Traumatic aneurysm:* Blunt trauma from outside producing wall injury or from intravascular interventions can be the cause for aneurysm formation.

Abdominal Aortic Aneurysm (Fig. 8.8)

Abdominal aorta is the most common site of aneurysm formation. It is three times more common in males and it is the disease of the old age, the frequency increases after 50

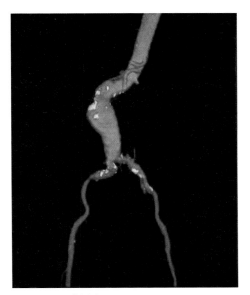

Fig. 8.8: CT angiogram of AAA

years of age. Many risk factors are associated with AAA like advanced age, male gender, hypertension, smoking, associated peripheral arterial disease, higher lipid level, COPD and positive family history. Chances of rupture of AAA are more in aged male, having history of smoking and of COPD.

Etiology and Pathogenesis

The AAA is said to be degenerative aneurysm due to atherosclerosis, but the etiology appears to be more complex involving many factors in combination. Aortic wall contains smooth muscle cells, matrix proteins, elastin and collagen arranged in organized, concentric manner to withstand pressure. Collagen gives strong support to prevent rupture and elastin resists dilatation. There is a progressive loss of elastin in the aortic aneurysm along with increase in metalloproteinase activity. This proteolysis occurring in media and inflammation are the important factors for developing AAA. Normal aortic wall contains 12% elastin, while it is only 1% in aneurysmal tissue. Shear stress near the aortic bifurcation, absence of vasa vasorum, etc. are thought to be additional factors. There is a sex-linked familial trend (autosomal recessive). Family members of female subject with AAA are more likely to have disease and first degree relatives are 11.6 times more likely to be affected as compared to general population. Smoking is a strong independent factor. Degenerative AAA accounts for >90% infrarenal AAA but other factors may be responsible in remaining cases, e.g. infection, connective tissue disorder, cystic medial necrosis, arteritis, trauma, anastomotic pseudoaneurysm, etc.

Natural History of AAA

On an average rate of expansion of AAA is 10% per year or 0.4 cm/year. Risk of rupture is related to the increasing diameter of the aneurysm. As per law of Laplace tensile strength of arterial wall is a function of pressure x radius. Consequently larger aneurysm is more likely to rupture. Aneurysm >5 cm diameter has an annual rate of rupture of 3-5%, 6 to 7 cm: 10-20%, 7 to 8 cm: 20-40%. Rapid expansion is associated with advanced age, smoking, hypertension, severe cardiac disease, stroke and high pulse pressure. Mortality of elective repair of AAA is 3-5%, while that of ruptured AAA is very significant >50%, which has not changed in decades. In females, even smaller aneurysms may rupture. Hence surgery or intervention is indicated early in AAA on elective basis. Sometimes layered thrombus may form inside aneurysm sac preventing expansion, but leading to frequent distal embolization.

Clinical Features

Most of the patients are asymptomatic and AAA is diagnosed accidentally if USG abdomen is done. Sometimes X-ray abdomen taken for some other purpose may show calcific aortic shadow. Patient may have vague abdominal pain due to stretching of surrounding or retroperitoneal tissue. Low back pain occurs due to erosion of vertebrae or even without erosion. Symptoms may occur due to ureteric compression, aortoenteric fistula (GI bleed), or lower limb ischemia due to embolization.

Examination in a thin built individual in a relaxed abdomen with knees flexed usually reveals pulsatile abdominal swelling to the left of umbilicus. Distal lower limb pulsations must be palpated and recorded as a guide for preoperative thrombotic occlusion or postoperative event causing absent pulses. Patient with ruptured AAA presents with acute abdominal pain, hypotension, shock and pulsatile abdominal mass.

Diagnosis

- *X-ray abdomen (plain):* It has a low sensitivity. Calcified wall of the aneurysm may be seen which may give clue to diagnosis in asymptomatic patient.

- *Duplex ultrasound (DUS):* This study of abdominal aorta is a good diagnostic and follow up modality. Size and extent of AAA can be judged fairly well. Intestinal gas shadows may interfere with good visualization.
- *CT scan with contrast enhancement:* It gives information about neck diameter, neck thrombosis, aneurysm diameter and length, distal extent into iliac arteries and patency of inferior mesenteric artery. 3-D reconstruction is very helpful for planning surgical as well as interventional approach.
- *Magnetic resonance imaging and angiography:* This is becoming popular as dye related complications are avoided, hence is useful in renally compromised patients also. Contraindications do exist and images are less clear.
- *Standard contrast angiography:* It is not routinely used presently as CTA and MRA give good information and are non- invasive. But this gives excellent visualization of AAA and in cases of accessory renal artery, horse-shoe kidney, mesenteric ischemia and lower limb ischemia. Usually prior to major intervention contrast angiography is desirable.
- Investigations for cardiac evaluation, renal functions, coagulation profile, pulmonary status and all routine tests required for a major surgery are carried out.

Medical Management

It is indicated for:
- Small AAA kept under surveillance
- For preoperative preparation of patients before intervention
- After the procedure some drugs are continued for short period and some lifelong.
- Patients with significant morbidity who are unfit for any interventions are kept on lifelong medications.

Medical treatment consists of antihypertensive therapy including beta blockers, lipid lowering drugs, antiplatelet drugs, drugs for cardiac disorder, control of blood sugar, and drugs for control of COPD, etc. Cessation of smoking is a must.

Surgical Treatment

Indications

- The AAA of size 5.5 cm or more must be electively repaired due to high incidence of rupture.
- In younger patient with AAA of size 4.5-5.5cm surgery may be considered keeping in view longevity and physical performance required at this age. Hence if the patient prefers early surgery after clear understanding of the disease, the same can be offered to such patient. It goes without saying that such a procedure should be performed by an experienced surgeon with very low mortality and excellent results.
- In females due to greater risk of rupture surgery can be offered for size 4.5-5cm.
- In elderly patients with decreased anticipated longevity due to associated comorbid conditions, when surgery is expected to be very high risk, balance should weigh in favor of conservative rather than operative treatment.
- Surgery is definitely indicated in ruptured AAA if the patient reaches the hospital in salvageable condition. The mortality is very high, but it is the only chance for the patient and must be availed.

Surgery—Approach and Details

- *Midline transperitoneal approach:* Laparotomy is done from xiphoid to pubic symphysis. It gives access to all abdominal contents, to aorta from supraceliac to both iliac arteries and hence it is a preferred approach by majority. Transverse colon is retracted upwards and small bowel is packed on right side. Thus root of mesentery and IV part of duodenum are exposed. The AAA exposed in its entire extent. Distal clamps are applied first after heparinization. Vertical clamp is applied 1.5-2 cm proximal to upper limit of aneurysm. Sac is incised, thrombus extracted and bleeding lumbar artery if any is transfixed. Inlay Dacron/ePTFE graft of appropriate size is sutured proximally with 4-0 Prolene and distally to iliac with 5-0 Prolene. Clamps are released sequentially avoiding embolization and sudden hypotension. Both femoral and sigmoid mesocolon pulsations are checked. Then sac is sutured over graft if the hemostasis is satisfactory.

- *Retroperitoneal approach:* This is preferred when there are intra- abdominal adhesions, stoma or patient has COPD. But it is difficult to reach right renal artery and distal right common iliac artery.

Complications of Surgery

i. Renal failure
ii. Lower limb ischemia
iii. Spinal cord ischemia
iv. Graft related delayed complications, such as graft infection, thrombosis, para-anastomotic pseudoaneurysm, and aorto-enteric fistula.

Results

Mortality rate in centers performing AAA surgery regularly is 2-4% and morbidity due to above mentioned causes is about 20%. In ruptured AAA mortality is 20-50%.

Endovascular Graft Repair of AAA

This is an innovation in which Dacron graft mounted on stent is deployed inside the aneurysm sac to exclude it from within, indications for the same are as follows:

- Anatomy of AAA should be suitable for endovascular graft repair of AAA (EVAR), i.e. it should not be tortuous and proximally neck of 1.5 cm at least should be available below renal artery level.
- In elderly patients with associated comorbid conditions and hostile abdomen, which precludes or makes surgery very high risk proposition, EVAR definitely needs to be considered as primary modality of treatment.
- Patient should be given idea about surgery and EVAR in details and the choice left to patient if both procedures appear suitable. If patient opts for EVAR it should definitely be offered.
- Patient who affords to pay for the cost of the procedure should be surely given benefit. But, in India, this modality is presently out of reach of majority due to cost factor.

Results

Mortality and morbidity are comparable with a surgical graft. If done in unsuitable patient rupture or other complication may necessitate conversion to open surgery with added complications. But pulmonary complications are less in EVAR. About 30-50% patients are being offered EVAR in developed countries. As endograft is inserted via arterial cut down limb ischemia needs to be meticulously watched. Complications like endoleak from lumbar arteries or IMA, renal toxicity due to contrast medium, graft thrombosis, etc. are all likely. Hence expertise is key to success, i.e. proper deployment of the endograft.

Other aneurysms like hepatic, splenic, femoral, popliteal, etc. are out of scope of this book. Enlargement of size above approximately 2 cm diameter is usual indication for intervention to prevent complications like thrombosis, embolization causing distal ischemia, rupture, etc.

Vascular Anomalies: Tumors and Malformations

Introduction

Treating physicians and vascular specialists are faced with the challenge of treating vascular anomalies, i.e. vascular tumors and malformations as their presentation is varied and incidence is rare, in contrast to well-defined lesions produced by atherosclerosis, peripheral arterial disease, venous thrombosis, aneurysms, etc. In addition, the difficulty is increased by confusing nomenclature of the disorders. International Society for Vascular Anomalies in 1996 suggested the term 'Vascular Anomalies' which are of two types: (1) vascular tumors and (2) vascular malformations. The term 'congenital' has been dropped as most of the lesions like infantile hemangiomas are not apparent at birth and others are present at cellular level only. As such, the term vascular malformation (VM) is descriptive enough. This also simplifies the nomenclature and avoids confusion in communication. Due to rarity of lesions and lack of comprehensive knowledge, many of the lesions were operated in past unnecessarily. With the recent information, the approach has drastically changed and surgical intervention has been advised rarely, other modalities with better results being available.

Embryology of Vascular Anomalies

Vascular system starts developing in the 3rd week of gestation and appears as network of interlacing blood spaces in the primitive mesenchyme. Three stages have been described:

Undifferentiated stage: Primitive blood spaces coalesce together into more organized capillary network. But arterial and venous systems are yet not differentiated. Arrest in this stage causes capillary malformation and peripheral vascular malformations.

Retiform stage: The capillary networks coalesce together in larger structures which are destined to become arteries and veins. Arrest or abnormality of this stage causes persistent embryonal veins and microfistulous arteriovenous malformations (AVM).

Maturation stage: The network matures and further differentiates into arterial and venous system. Capillary network of stage I continue in adult life. Macrofistulous AVMs of named branches, popliteal vein aneurysm, persistent sciatic artery, etc. occur due to anomalies of stage III.

Incidence

Vascular anomaly (VA), particularly VM includes lesions, which may involve arteries, veins, capillaries and lymphatics in varying proportions. The VMs constitute 48% (nearly half), arteriovenous malformations (AVMs) 36% (nearly 1/3rd). Mixed lesions constitute 15% and pure arterial defects are rare about 1%.

Hamburg Classification

Hamburg classification was approved by experts in the meeting held at Hamburg, Germany. This has proposed four main groups like arterial, venous, arteriovenous and mixed. The lesions involving axial/central vessels are called truncular and the ones involving peripheral vessels are called extratruncular. Truncular could be obstructive or dilating, i.e. aneurysmal and extratruncular could be localized or diffuse.

Vascular Tumors

Infantile hemangioma (IH) is the most common tumor in children occurring in 4-10% neonates of white race and is less common in African and Asian infants. It is more common in girls, occurs as a single mass but about 20% may appear at multiple sites like skin, liver, gastrointestinal tract and brain. It appears about 2 weeks after birth as pale or red spot. Then there is a rapid growth in next 1 year in proliferating phase when it appears as a firm, tense and noncompressible mass. Superficial veins are seen radiating from tumor. Ulceration may occur especially on lips, anogenital region and limbs. During next 5-7 years the mass regresses significantly and by the age of 12 years only redundant skin and fibrofatty tissue may remain.

Hepatic IH is variable in size from tiny asymptomatic nodule to large or multiple masses and is more common in girls. Usually they present at the age of 1-16 weeks of infancy due to hepatomegaly, anemia and congestive heart failure.

Histologically, the IH shows features specific to the stage. In proliferating stage, they have actively dividing endothelial cells, basement membrane is multilaminated and there are abundant mast cells (features which are not present in venous malformations). Involuting IH have flat endothelial cells, vascular thrombosis and fibrofatty tissue.

Differential Diagnosis

1. Lymphatic malformation
2. Venous malformation
3. Pyogenic granuloma.

Diagnosis

Duplex Ultrasound

Differentiates deep IH from VM, shows dense parenchyma and fast flow in proliferating phase. It also shows decreased arterial resistance and increased venous velocity. Duplex ultrasound (DUS) is also helpful to diagnose intrahepatic (IH).

MRI

It is quite helpful to diagnose IH, which is seen as a solid mass. Flow voids within and around mass indicates A-V shunting between feeding arteries and dilated draining veins. During involuted phase it is seen as vascular fatty mass. Intracranial IH are easily diagnosed on MRI.

Treatment

Most IH regress by the age of 7 years or up to extended period of 12 years. Hence, the child must be kept under observation. Those around vital structures like airway, eyes, or those growing rapidly need prompt attention. Following modalities are available.

Conservative

Ulceration and bleeding should be managed with antibiotics, daily dressing with topical lidocaine, hydrocolloid and antibiotic ointment. Compression stops the bleeding and occasionally a stitch may be required. Ulcer may heal within days to few weeks.

Drugs Therapy

About 10% IH may produce life-threatening complications especially in cervicofacial region. Ocular and airway compression by subglottic IH, gastrointestinal tract bleeding and high output congestive heart failure are the issues, which need to be addressed on emergency basis.

Intralesional corticosteroid injection: Therapy is indicated in small, localized cutaneous IH located on nasal tip, lip, eyelid, or extremity which has been shown to decrease proliferation and tumor mass. Triamcinolone 2-3 mg/kg body weight is injected intralesionally with 26G needle slowly. Systemic embolization is prevented by finger compression at periphery and in extremity by tourniquet. Compression if possible like in extremity, is maintained. Three sessions at the interval of 6-8 weeks are usually required.

Systemic corticosteroids: Prednisolone 2-3 mg/kg of body weight is given in the morning. Response occurs usually within 1 week. Then, the dose is tapered every 2-4 weeks and maintained till the age of 10-11 months. The therapy is indicated for large masses and compression of vital structures as mentioned above. About 20-30% fail to respond to corticosteroid therapy.

Interferon (IFN) alpha-2a or -2b is indicated when there is no response to corticosteroid therapy or complications occur or prolonged course is required. The IFN is used alone in the dose of 2-3 million units per square meter of body surface subcutaneously daily for 6-12 months in endangering or life-threatening IH. It is effective in more than 80% of tumors, which fail to respond to corticosteroids. During therapy hepatic enzymes are raised and neurological complications like spastic diplegia may occur.

Note: Cytotoxic drugs like vincristine, cyclophosphamide have been tried to avoid neurologic complications produced by IFN.

Embolization Therapy

It is advised when corticosteroid therapy fails and in severe congestive heart failure which occurs usually due to hepatic tumor. Embolization here is used to occlude large percentage of arterio- venous shunts.

Laser Therapy

Its routine use is not recommended because it is used in superficial IH which otherwise also regress with age. Only indications for Laser photocoagulations are:

a. Persistent telangiectasia after involution phase
b Unilateral subglottic IH in proliferating phase
c. Laser therapy at 4-6 week intervals helps in ulcer healing in ulcerated and bleeding IH.

Surgery

Indications:

a. Well-localized, pedunculated IH particularly if it is ulcerated and bleeding repeatedly.
b. IH of upper eyelid which does not regress with corticosteroid therapy, which should be resected or debulked.
c. GI tract hemangiomas which bleed repeatedly despite drugs can be excised by enterotomy or by endoscopic approach.
d. After involution if large fibrofatty mass or bulky skin is left resection is advised.

Vascular Malformations

Faulty development at some stage of vasculogenesis causes VM. It may be of any type, e.g. capillary, venous, arterial, lymphatic or mixed. Most of them are sporadic but some are inherited.

Capillary Malformation

It can be localized, extensive or rarely multiple, composed of mainly capillary sized vessels, which sometimes may consist of even venular size vessels. It is placed in superficial dermis and nerve fibers are scanty in the surrounding tissue. It can occur anywhere in the body but when occurs on face it is obvious.

The usual location is superficial where it appears pink and becomes nodular later. Often overgrowth of soft tissue and skeleton occurs in the affected area, which may produce limb size disparity. Overlying CM may also indicate possibility of underlying structural abnormality, e.g. spina bifida, encephalocele, etc.

Treatment: Laser therapy is successful in nearly 70% cases of CMs. Small fibrofatty nodules can be excised. Facial soft tissue or skeletal overgrowth can be surgically corrected.

Lymphatic Malformation

Lymphatic malformations (LMs) are composed of vascular spaces filled with protein rich fluid and eosinophils, lymphocytes and skeletal and smooth muscle cells form the wall. The LMs are usually noticed at birth or before 2 years of age. They may occur as localized spongy lesions or as diffuse lesions and may involve internal organs. Two types are recognized:
1. Microcystic (lymphangioma)
2. Macrocystic (cystic hygroma).

These two types may also occur in various combinations. Most common locations are axilla, chest, cervicofacial region, mediastinum, retroperitoneum, etc. Overlying skin in superficial lesions could be puckered and bluish. Intravascular bleed may occur. Localized soft tissue overgrowth may occur causing disfigurement or compression, which produces symptoms depending on location.

Diagnosis

- Ultrasonography confirms macrocystic LM.
- Magnetic resonance imaging shows LMs as hyperintense on T2-weighted sequences due to high water content. The MR lymphangiography shows dilated or interrupted lymphatics, especially in limbs.

Treatment

This is required usually for secondary infection causing cellulitis and for bleeding inside LM. Intralymphatic bleed causes pain which can be managed with antibiotics, analgesics and compression in suitable locations. Sclerotherapy with pure ethanol, sodium tetradecyl sulfate or doxycycline is advised in macrocystic LM. Resection offers the potential chance for cure, but total excision is rarely possible. Damage to vital structures must be meticulously avoided. Repeat surgery may be required in some cases. Repeated postoperative aspirations of fluid help in some patients to avoid recurrence. Recurrence rate is 40% after incomplete resection and 17% after complete excision as judged during operation on gross findings.

Venous Malformations

This is the most common congenital vascular anomaly, which is usually solitary and present at birth but clinically not appreciated easily. It appears as soft and bluish compressible swelling. Most common location is skin and subcutaneous tissue but involvement of muscles, viscera and central nervous system is possible. The VM grows with the child and phleboliths may form by 2 years of age. Further growth occurs at puberty. The child may experience more pain and stiffness after morning awakening which is a typical feature. Soft tissue overgrowth may occur causing various presentations depending on location. In bowel, it may produce intermittent bleed. If child presents with multiple VMs, familial transmission should be considered and in this category glomuvenous malformation (GVM) is the most common form, which presents as large clusters or nodules involving extremities. This is tender on palpation but painless on morning awakening unlike common VM and it does not respond to compression garments.

Diagnosis

The MRI is the best modality to diagnose VM. It is hyperintense on T2-weighted images and contrast enhancement differentiates it from LM. Phleboliths and thrombi are seen on MR venography which is a helpful study for large extremity VMs. Rarely, the direct contrast venography may be required for evaluation.

Coagulation profile should be studied. Usually prothrombin time is increased, APTT is normal, fibrinogen level is low and D-dimer is increased. Platelet count is low (30000-50000).

Treatment

This is indicated for pain, cosmetic appearance and functional disturbances. For extremity VMs elastic compression stockings are helpful. Thrombosed veins, which cause pain respond to aspirin in low dose, i.e. 75 mg daily or on alternate days. Definitive treatment is as follows:

Sclerotherapy: Small cutaneous or oral/mucosal VMs can be treated with dilute 100% ethanol or sodium tetradecyl sulfate 1%. Larger ones can be treated by sclerotherapy preferably under anesthesia and under USG guidance. Systemic spread of sclerosant is prevented by some compression around. Repeat sessions at roughly bimonthly intervals may be required.

Local complications like blisters, cutaneous necrosis and nerve injury may occur. Systemic embolization may produce hemolysis, renal damage, anaphylaxis or sudden cardiac arrest. Recurrence to some extent occurs in many cases, but the size of VM is definitely reduced.

Resection:
a. Small localized VM
b. Larger ones can be resected after reducing size by laser or sclerotherapy.
c. Full thickness GI VM needs bowel resection. Resection should be conservative. Endoscopic resection is possible in approachable areas.

d. Diffuse colorectal, pelvic VMs are best left alone unless bleeding forces some intervention to be carried out. Then sclerotherapy and bowel diversion may be of help.

Arteriovenous Malformations (Figs 9.1A and B)

The AVMs can occur at various locations like skin, liver, brain, lungs, etc. Skin AVM is present at birth and may be mistaken for infantile hemangioma due to firm bluish appearance. But

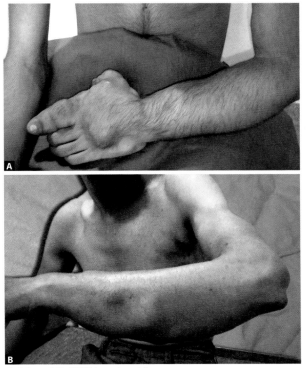

Figs 9.1A and B: AVM hand and forearm

in later life appearance becomes clear, as due to minor trauma or during puberty due to hormonal changes the size of AVM enlarges and mass appears beneath the superficial stain on skin. There is a local warmth, thrill and radiating prominent veins from the periphery of the mass. Later on complications like infection, pain, ulceration, ischemia and bleeding may occur. Lower limb AVM may develop curious dry plaque on the surface. Larger AVMs can produce major arteriovenous shunting producing congestive heart failure. Various stages of AVMs are described by Schobinger as follows:

Stage I (quiescence): Pink blue stain, warmth and AV shunting

Stage II (expansion): Stage I + size increased, thrill/bruit, tortuous veins

Stage III (destruction): Stage II + skin dystrophy, ulcer, bleed, persistent pain and tissue necrosis

Stage IV (decompensation): Stage III + cardiac failure
(adapted from Rutherford's Vascular Surgery Textbook, sixth edition, volume two).

Diagnosis

Duplex ultrasound usually confirms diagnosis. The MRI with MR angiography is the best investigation to confirm diagnosis, to describe the extent and blood flow pattern to the AVM (Fig. 9.2).

Treatment

Usually no treatment is required during infancy or childhood. However, localized AVM can be resected fully, which avoids future complications. Stage I AVM can be excised. Complications like ulceration, bleeding, ischemia (stage III) or CHF (stage IV) necessitate intervention. Superselective arterial embolization is helpful to reduce size and to stop bleeding. Surgical resection should be carried out within 24-72 hours after embolization.

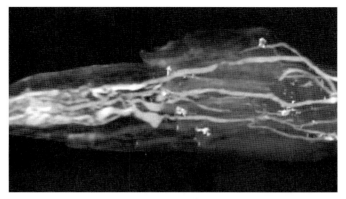

Fig. 9.2: MRA of AVM hand and forearm

Complete excision, however, cannot be guaranteed. If access is difficult due to tortuous feeder artery, size of AVM can be reduced by sclerotherapy through nidus (center) of AVM. However, this requires expertise and experience to carry out Sclerotherapy in the presence of arterial feeders. Systemic embolization must be prevented by compression at its periphery. However, neurological and soft tissue damage is likely.

Axial or major artery of the area involved must not be embolized, sclerosed or ligated as this leads to recruitment of additional feeders and further embolization is not possible due to 'no access'. In the areas, which are not accessible surgically, embolization and palliative treatment is only possible.

Mixed VMs

Various combinations of venous, arterial, capillary and lymphatics have been described, which may have slow or fast flow through AV shunts. Most of them are managed conservatively. Other treatment modalities are employed like

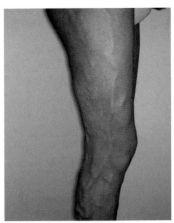

Fig. 9.3: Venous anomaly—Klippel-Trenaunay syndrome

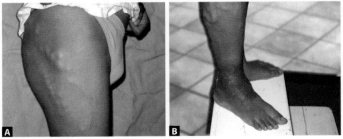

Figs 9.4A and B: Venous anomaly

they are used in other malformations. Examples of these are Klippel-Trenaunay (KT) syndrome (slow flow) and Parkes Weber syndrome (fast flow) (Figs 9.3 and 9.4).

Carotid Artery Occlusive Disease

An occlusive disease at the origin of internal carotid artery is the most common cause of cerebrovascular accidents or stroke. Stroke may produce paralysis, aphasia, blindness and weakness of limbs, which can really be debilitating. The affected person may become burden on the family and may also become psychologically crippled due to this dependence. Thus stroke produces enormous burden on the economic status of the health care system. Hence prevention of cerebrovascular accidents, treatment of occlusive disease of carotid arteries in particular, will remain an important health care issue.

Some definitions must be understood before while treating carotid artery occlusive disease (CAOD).

Stroke

It is also called focal cerebral ischemic disease, which indicates loss of cerebral function lasting more than 24 hours and occurs due to ischemic vascular etiology. Incidence of stroke in general population is 0.2% per annum which rises with advancing age. It could be about 2% above the age of 80 years.

Transient Ischemic Attack

Transient ischemic attack (TIA) is defined as a stroke lasting less than 24 hours. In fact many TIA's recover within few minutes. Sometimes TIA lasts longer than 24 hours and recovers within 3 weeks, which is called "reversible ischemic neurological deficit" (RIND).

Pathogenesis of Stroke and TIA

Carotid Artery Thrombosis

It occurs due to atherosclerosis at carotid artery bifurcation and involves internal carotid artery (ICA) and is responsible for more than 80% of all the strokes. Because it is a gradual process collateral circulation develops among arteries of circle of Willis, which prevents occurrence of stroke and the patient may remain asymptomatic. If thrombus propagation stops before origin of ophthalmic artery, chances of stroke are much less. If it propagates beyond ophthalmic artery into middle cerebral artery territory anything from TIA to stroke may occur.

Hypoperfusion

Beyond stenosed carotid circulation decrease in perfusion pressure may occur, e.g. due to cardiac event causing arrhythmia and hypotension. Especially when the collateral circulation is not adequately developed, such an event can cause stroke or TIA. Hypoperfusion is responsible for cerebral event in about 15% cases.

Cardiogenic Embolization

This is responsible for about 10% cases. Emboli may arise from native valve vegetations, prosthetic valve vegetations, atrial myxoma, and mural thrombus from LV myocardial infarct or from LV aneurysm. Emboli from major aortic arch and arch arteries are atherosclerotic in origin and contain platelets, cholesterol, calcific debris, etc. which may lodge in cerebral circulation.

Hematological Disorders

About 5% of the strokes are caused due to hypercoagulable state induced by polycythemia, sickle cell disease, leukemia, malignancy, thrombocytosis, lupus anticoagulant, deficiency of protein C and S and of antithrombin III.

Rare Causes

Migraine, oral contraceptives, Takayasu's arteritis, giant cell arteritis, SLE, radiation induced arteritis, fibromuscular dysplasia, carotid artery kinks, aneurysms and coils, carotid body tumor, trauma, etc. are rare causes of cerebrovascular accidents being responsible for about 5% cases.

Diagnosis

Complete neurological examination is important to record the deficit which may point to possible area of involvement. Similarly cardiac examination could indicate possible causes as already mentioned. Association of peripheral arterial disease again should be evaluated as it may modify the plan of treatment. Bruit on carotid artery must be specially looked for (Carotid bruit appears when carotid arterial luminal diameter is reduced at least by 50%).

Duplex ultrasound with color Doppler scan is an important modality to diagnose CAOD. It gives location of narrowing, type of plaque, velocity of flow and luminal diameter narrowing. Transcranial Doppler has low frequency probe which can study intracranial brain circulation across the skull bones.

Magnetic resonance imaging (MRI) with magnetic resonance angiography (MRA) is a very sensitive and specific investigation for stroke patients. Its advantage is that it can be done in renally compromised patients and is more sensitive in diagnosing acute cerebral injury. MRA gives complete outline of circulation in the circle of Willis like narrowing, occlusion, extent, collateral circulation. Intracranial extension is a difficult disease to manage; hence the extent of the disease must be exactly mapped (Fig. 10.1).

Traditional carotid angiography done by puncturing carotid artery is rarely used these days.

Apart from diagnostic investigations as above, kidney function tests, blood sugar level, lipid profile, thrombophilia profile, ECG, etc. must be carried out for planning comprehensive management.

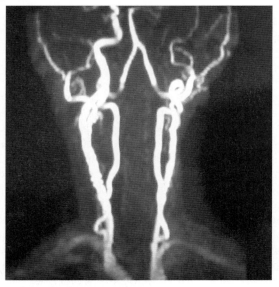

Fig. 10.1: Carotid MR angiography

Medical Management of CAOD

Medical treatment for hypertension, antiplatelet drugs like aspirin and clopidogrel, statins to reduce cholesterol all these modify the clinical status of the patient. European Carotid Surgery Trial (ECST) has established that surgery and medical treatment combined has better clinical outcome than medical treatment alone in the management of CAOD.

Surgical treatment of carotid stenosis has been suggested by both ECST and North American Symptomatic Carotid Endarterectomy Trial (NASCET) for 70-99% stenosis. Asymptomatic Carotid Atherosclerosis Study (ACAS) has established the role of carotid endarterectomy in asymptomatic patient having >60% stenosis, as it was found to reduce stroke rate by 50%.

Thus indications of CEA are:

- TIA
- RIND
- Stroke which has recovered satisfactorily
- Asymptomatic CAOD with more than 70% stenosis.

Contraindications

1. Acute stroke
2. Stroke with significant residual deficit
3. Total or 100% carotid occlusion
4. Significant comorbid conditions like advanced malignancy or heart disease, etc.

Surgical Technique

Anesthesia

Regional anesthesia is preferred by some surgeons as the patient is awake and any neurological deficit during surgery can be identified on table. But anxious patients may not cooperate.

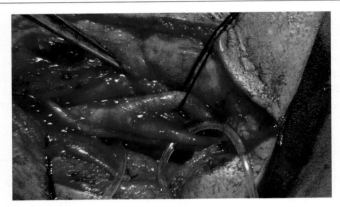

Fig. 10.2: Carotid bifurcation

General anesthesia (GA) keeps the patient immobile and free of anxiety. Any vascular event or bleed causing hypotension can be better managed. But fitness for GA requires many investigations and strict criteria.

Technique: With support under the shoulder neck is turned to opposite side. Incision is taken along the anterior border of sternomastoid muscle and deepened. Common facial vein is ligated and divided from internal jugular vein and common carotid; internal carotid artery (ICA) and external carotid artery (ECA) are gently mobilized and taped (Fig. 10.2). Excess handling of these arteries is avoided. Injection heparin is given intravenously. Common carotid artery (CCA), ICA and ECA are gently clamped and distal ICA stump pressure is recorded. If it is > 25 mm Hg, ICA can be safely clamped; otherwise intracarotid shunt is inserted. Vertical incision is taken on CCA and extended on ICA beyond palpable thrombus. Thrombus is carefully dissected with intima and sharply cut off at junction with normal shining inner wall of CCA and ICA (Figs 10.3 and 10.4). The interior of CCA and ICA are thoroughly flushed with

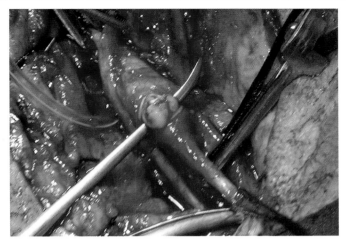

Fig. 10.3: Carotid endarterectomy—thrombus in carotid artery

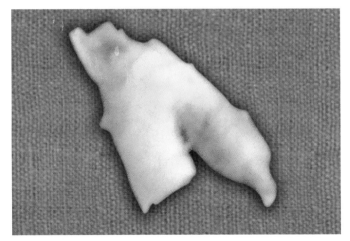

Fig. 10.4: Carotid endarterectomy—removed thrombus

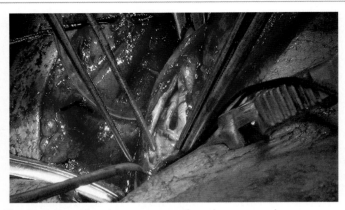

Fig. 10.5: Carotid endarterectomy—thrombus removed

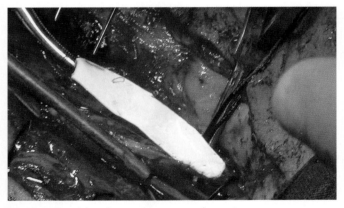

Fig. 10.6: Carotid endarterectomy—patch repair

heparinized saline (Fig. 10.5). If ICA is hypoplastic, arteriotomy is closed with PTFE or vein patch. Finally clamps are released (Fig. 10.6).

Complications:
1. Perioperative stroke
2. Cranial nerve injury occurs in about 30% patients.
3. Recurrent carotid stenosis can occur in about 30% cases which is mild and patients are usually asymptomatic. Only 3% patients are symptomatic requiring intervention.

Carotid Artery Stenting

It is a catheter-based intervention wherein using balloon the stenosis is dilated and stent is implanted. To prevent intracerebral embolization distal protection device is used. The procedure is costly and long-term results are awaited. It is presently indicated in patients in whom surgery is risky.

Carotid Body Tumor

History

In 1743: Von Haller first described carotid body.
In 1880: Reigner tried first resection but patient died.
In 1886: Maydl did first resection but patient developed hemiplegia and aphasia.
In 1903: Scudder did first successful resection.

Incidence

Exact incidence of carotid body tumor (CBT) is difficult to quote because the tumor is rare and only small number of cases has been studied. Approximate incidence is 0.5% of all tumors. Male to female sex ratio is also not clear, while in some series females predominate. It is more common in people living at high altitude. Most of them become clinically overt in 5th decade, while any age above 2nd decade is affected. So far more than 900 cases have been described in the literature.

Physiology

Carotid body is approximately of $5 \times 3 \times 2$ mm in size of the size of grain of wheat, located at common carotid artery bifurcation on posterior medial surface in adventitia to which it is attached by Meyer's ligament, also carrying its blood supply. It has very high blood flow and oxygen consumption, approximately 0.2 L/gm/min (more than that of heart and brain). It is reddish brown in color. It is derived from mesodermal and neural crest elements. The tumor arising from it is called paraganglioma because it arises from autonomic paraganglion cells.

The tumor is composed of mainly two types of cells:

1. Type I, i.e. chief cells which have granular, eosinophilic cytoplasm and they secrete catecholamines.
2. Type II cells are 'sustentacular cells' which are supporting cells.

The tumors are very vascular and clusters of cell balls called 'Zellballen' are seen between capillaries.

Function of Carotid Body

It acts through autonomic control. It responds to decrease in oxygen in circulating blood and to lesser extent to increase in circulating CO_2 and decrease in pH of circulating blood. It responds by increasing respiratory rate, heart rate and blood pressure through chief cells. Carotid body also responds to stimulus by increased blood temperature.

Pathology

The tumors occur in neck, at base of skull, in nasopharynx and throughout body cavities and are well-circumscribed, rubbery and reddish brown. There is no true capsule. The tumor grows and splays the common carotid artery bifurcation. It extends towards the base of skull. Nerve supply of the carotid body is through glossopharyngeal nerve. Carotid body tumors are of two types:

1. *Nonchromaffin type:* Which form 95% of the group and these tumors do not secrete catecholamines.

2. *Chromaffin paraganglioma:* This is rare and hormone secreting tumor. However 60% of the retroperitoneal tumors secrete catecholamines.

Two subtypes of each have been described:

i. Sporadic form is more common and about 5% of them could have bilateral tumors.

ii. Familial form is not common and transmission is by autosomal dominant pattern. More than 30% of them may have bilateral tumors and screening of family members has been advised to diagnose the mass when it is small in size and easy to excise.

Incidence of malignancy is variable from 2-50% and is controversial. Malignant potential can be judged by spread to regional lymph nodes or distant metastases to kidney, thyroid, lungs, bones, etc. These tumors are usually slow growing for many years, but they can produce disability and death even without malignancy. Mortality without surgery is about 8%.

Clinical Presentation

Most commonly the mass remains unnoticed for a long time before the patient seeks medical attention. Usual presentation is a nodule in the neck near angle of mandible in nearly 75% patients. There could be nonspecific symptoms like pain in the nodule and in the neck, headache, dizziness, tinnitus, hoarseness, syncope, etc. As about 5% tumors may be hormonally active, they may present with flushing, palpitation, arrhythmia, photophobia, sweating, associated with headache and syncope. Rarely symptoms related to dysfunction of cranial nerves like vagus, hypoglossal and cervical sympathetic nerves may occur.

Examination of neck reveals a mass located near angle of mandible, mobile horizontally but not vertically due to its attachment to carotid bifurcation. It is usually rubbery, firm and noncompressible. Rarely may it be bilateral. Usually transmitted pulsations are clearly palpable and bruit may be heard. Very rarely signs due to compression of vagus, hypoglossal nerves and sympathetic chain may be demonstrated. Clinical examination is important to assess the extent of the mass for planning of surgical excision, as bigger the mass more technically difficult it is for excision.

Diagnosis

- Duplex ultrasound is a very useful modality which is being used most commonly for the diagnosis of CBT. It gives information about the size of the mass, its relation to carotid bifurcation and hypervascularity. Associated atherosclerotic or aneurysmal changes in carotid arteries can also be documented.

- Both CT and MRI help in demonstrating size, extent of the tumor. Rapid sequence CT can differentiate aneurysm from tumor, while MRI with MR angiography is superior to demonstrate vascularity, relation of the tumor to surrounding structures, which is important for surgical planning. Complete cerebral circulation can be studied. Overall MRI is a better modality to evaluate CBT (Fig. 11.1).

- Contrast angiography is rarely done and is helpful for demonstrating splaying of carotid bifurcation by tumor mass (Lyre sign), its complete vascular supply which is useful for preoperative embolization in very vascular and large tumor.

- Needle aspiration biopsy or wedge biopsy are specifically mentioned here not to be carried out due to danger of massive hemorrhage.

- Routine estimation of catecholamines and their byproducts in urine (VMA) is not advised. Only in cases with clinical suspicion of hormonal activity the same is done.

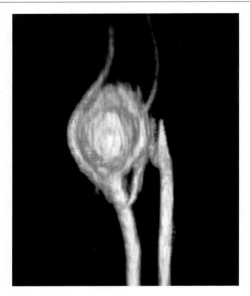

Fig. 11.1: MRA of carotid body tumor

Shamblin's Anatomical Groups of CBT

Based on investigation as above CBTs can be divided in three groups based on the criteria described by Shamblin and his colleagues from Mayo clinic:

- *Group I (26%):* Small tumor, minimally attached to carotid artery, easy to excise.
- *Group II (46%):* Larger tumor, partly surround the carotids, can be resected but intraluminal shunt may be required.
- *Group III (27%):* Very large tumors encasing carotids, arterial resection and grafting required.

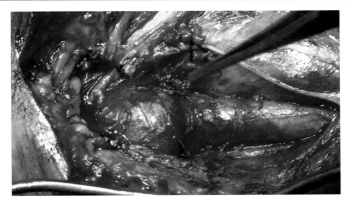

Fig. 11.2: Carotid body tumor—Exposed

Treatment

Surgery remains the best treatment in carotid body tumor (Figs 11.2 to 11.6). Being very vascular, technically difficult tumor to excise when large, surgery is advised when it is small and easily resectable (Shamblin I). General anesthesia and nasotracheal intubation is preferred. Tumor is exposed by an oblique incision along with anterior border of sternomastoid muscle. Common, external and internal arteries are taped. Tumor is mobilized in subadventitial plane controlling bleeding carefully at every step. Gentle handling is required to avoid arrhythmias and hypertension. Surrounding nerves also must be carefully protected. In Shamblin type II sometimes carotid shunt may be required and in type III excision and interposition graft may be required. In larger tumors subluxation of temporomandibular joint may be required. Sometimes ECA may need ligation and is of no consequence but if ICA needs ligation, stroke may occur.

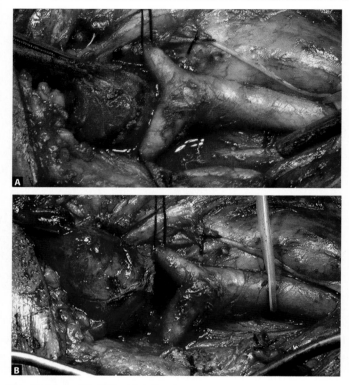

Figs 11.3A and B: CBT—Mobilized

Results of Surgery

External carotid artery (ECA) ligation is harmless. Incidence of stroke could be 20-50% if ICA has been ligated. Cranial nerve injury has been seen in about 20% patients of various degrees. In long-term results, survival is comparable to general population. Recurrence rate is <6% after resection and metastases occur in <2% cases.

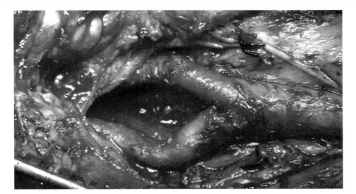

Fig. 11.4: Carotid body tumor—removed—note carotid bifurcation

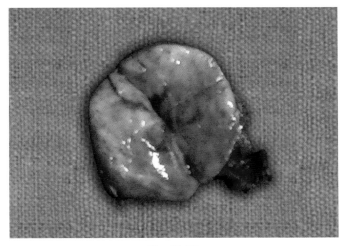

Fig. 11.5A

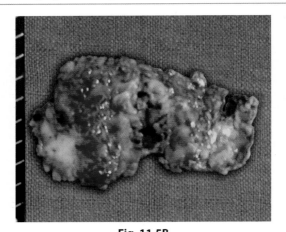

Fig. 11.5B
Figs 11.5A and B: Carotid body tumor—Specimen cut

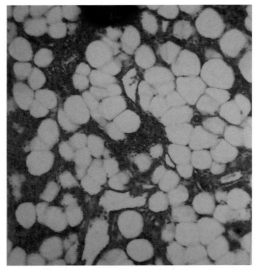

Fig. 11.6: Carotid body tumor—Histopathology

Other treatment modalities: Preoperative radiotherapy has not been found to be effective. However in large tumors with malignant potential radiotherapy gives additional relief. There is no role of chemotherapy. Preoperative embolization of the tumor has been advocated by some to reduce vascularity, but thrombosis of ICA and cerebral embolization has been reported.

Mesenteric Occlusive Disease

Introduction

Mesenteric ischemia is a vascular disease having very high mortality ranging from 50 to 75%. Delay in diagnosis and treatment are the main contributing factors in high mortality rate. As the clinical picture of 'Acute Abdomen' is similar in ischemic and nonischemic bowel conditions, it is difficult to point out mesenteric occlusive disease as the cause for such presentation. Incidence is rising due to increased longevity of the population and better awareness amongst treating physicians about this entity. Early diagnosis is essential and treatment must be initiated before irreversible bowel ischemia occurs.

About 6-10% of autopsies show approximately 50% involvement of at least one of the three major mesenteric vessels. Out of the patients undergoing aortography for peripheral arterial disease about 27% showed more than 50% stenosis of celiac and superior mesenteric arteries.

Blood Supply of Bowel (Fig. 12.1)

Celiac artery (CA), superior mesenteric artery (SMA) and inferior mesenteric artery (IMA) are the three major arteries supplying blood to intestine. The CA supplies blood to foregut and

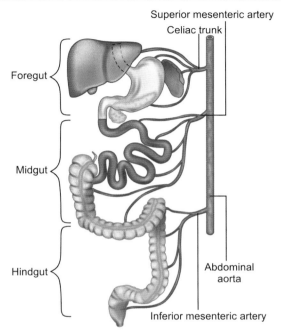

Fig. 12.1: Blood supply of gut

stomach up to second part of duodenum. The SMA supplies blood beyond second part of duodenum up to right two-thirds of transverse colon. The hindgut from distal third of transverse colon to rectum is supplied by IMA. Pancreaticoduodenal arcade forms anastomosis between CA and SMA and marginal artery of Drummond and Riolan arc between SMA and IMA. These collateral arteries are insufficient and inconstant to supply blood to intestine in case of acute or chronic occlusion of mesenteric arteries.

Types of Mesenteric Occlusive Disease

Four types of MOD are recognized:
1. Acute embolic mesenteric ischemia—Most common
2. Acute thrombotic mesenteric ischemia
3. Chronic mesenteric ischemia
4. Nonobstructive mesenteric ischemia (NOMI).

In addition about 20% develop mesenteric venous thrombosis.

The SMA is the most commonly involved vessel in acute occlusion. In patient of atherosclerosis of mesenteric arteries acute thrombotic occlusion of SMA may occur. Usually origin of the artery is involved and collaterals are spared. Acute embolic occlusion occurs from emboli from native cardiac valves, implanted artificial valves, mural thrombi, in atrial fibrillation, etc. In nonobstructive mesenteric ischemia or NOMI otherwise normal mesenteric blood flow is present and ischemia occurs due to low flow state. Element of spasm is important. In chronic occlusion due to atherosclerosis, the process is longstanding and typically two of three major mesenteric arteries are involved.

Rare causes of mesenteric ischemia:
- Median arcuate ligament syndrome—Here during expiration CA is compressed extrinsically near diaphragmatic hiatus due to arcuate ligament of diaphragm.
- Ligation of IMA during abdominal aortic surgery, mesenteric ischemia develops if collaterals are inadequate.
- Dissection of abdominal aorta involving mesenteric arteries.
- Rare causes like radiation arteritis, nonspecific mesenteric arteritis, cholesterol emboli, etc.

Clinical Features

Typical presentation of MOD is abdominal pain disproportionate to the clinical findings, which occurs due to acute embolic or thrombotic mesenteric occlusion involving SMA. Male to female ratio is 1:3 and usual age group is 40-70 years. Patient may have underlying cardiac disease, atrial fibrillation or atherosclerotic process. Following abdominal pain, later in course of the disease patient develops bloody diarrhea due to sloughing of ischemic mucosa. Nausea, vomiting, fever and abdominal distension are common but nonspecific manifestations. Diffuse abdominal tenderness, guarding and rigidity are signs of bowel infarction and are usually bad prognostic signs.

In chronic atherosclerotic occlusion symptoms are insidious and 70% have chronic abdominal angina usually precipitated by any illness producing dehydration due to diarrhea or vomiting. If not recognized in time clinical picture may worsen causing progressive abdominal distension, oliguria, severe metabolic acidosis, etc.

In NOMI pain is present in 70% patients. It is usually severe, may vary in location, intensity and character. If there is no pain, silent bowel ischemia is suggested by progressive abdominal distension with acidosis. Diagnosis of NOMI should be entertained in elderly patient with congestive heart failure, acute myocardial infarction with cardiogenic shock, hypovolemic or hemorrhagic shock, sepsis, pancreatitis, patient on digitalis or on vasopressors like epinephrine.

Diagnosis

Routine Investigations

These are done for general evaluation of the status of the patient. Hemoglobin and blood counts are done because hemoconcentration and leukocytosis may be present. Renal function tests and electrolyte estimation are important for assessment of renal status, and hyperkalemia and azotemia are present in late bowel ischemia. Increased serum amylase and LDH are nonspecific parameters. Metabolic acidosis may be present due to anaerobic metabolism. Doxylase 25 gm is given orally to differentiate malabsorption syndrome from MOD. Urine sample is tested for doxylase excretion. In malabsorption syndrome 5 gm is excreted within next 5 hours.

Plain X-ray Abdomen (Erect Film)

It is important to exclude bowel perforation, obstruction or volvulus. Paralytic ileus with gasless abdomen is common finding in acute mesenteric ischemia.

2D Echo

Source of emboli from heart as well as ischemic heart disease, congestive failure can be diagnosed on 2D echocardiography.

Duplex Ultrasound

It is useful screening modality. It can give clue to mesenteric artery stenosis. If peak systolic velocity for SMA is >275 cm/ sec and for CA it is > 200 cm/sec it indicates more than 70% stenosis. Reversal of blood flow in hepatic or splenic artery gives indirect clue to the major arterial stenosis.

Magnetic Resonance Angiography

It gives important information about arterial circulation and can be used in patients with deranged renal function. Venous phase study gives information about venous circulation in splanchnic bed and helps in diagnosis of mesenteric vein thrombosis. Pancreatic and other visceral pathology can be detected.

Contrast Angiography (Fig. 12.2)

It should be performed in a suspected case of MOD for early diagnosis. It shows CA/SMA occlusion/stenosis at/near origin from aorta. The IMA is usually found already occluded in majority. Four types of mesenteric occlusive diseases as already

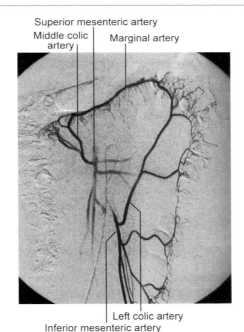

Superior mesenteric artery
Middle colic artery
Marginal artery
Left colic artery
Inferior mesenteric artery

Fig. 12.2: Marginal artery between superior mesenteric artery and inferior mesenteric artery

described can be differentiated which is very important for planning management. In embolic SMA occlusion 'meniscus sign' is positive due to embolus lodgement in middle colic artery branch of SMA, showing normal proximal SMA and then abrupt cut off. Mesenteric thrombosis in contrast occurs in most proximal part of SMA and gradually tapers off for 1-2 cm. Collateral circulation is seen in chronic MOD and in NOMI relatively normal SMA is seen, along with segmental vasospasm. Catheter directed vasodilator and papaverine therapy is indicated if diagnosis of NOMI is established. Thrombolytic therapy in chronic occlusion is not very encouraging and is required for prolonged period.

Treatment

Patient should be intensively monitored. Central venous catheter is inserted for drugs, fluid supplement and venous pressure monitoring. Arterial pressure is monitored by putting arterial line. Foley's catheter is inserted for urine output record. Higher antibiotics are started along with anticoagulant like heparin. It is desirable to obtain angiogram to confirm diagnosis and to plan type of surgical procedure. However, if patient has signs of acute abdomen and is taken for surgery immediately, this advantage may not be available. Then mesenteric arterial occlusion is intraoperative diagnosis.

In acute embolic mesenteric occlusion, midline laparotomy is done. The SMA is exposed by mobilizing and retracting medially 4th part of duodenum. By horizontal arteriotomy embolectomy is done using Fogarty balloon catheter and intestinal viability is assessed. Nonviable bowel must be resected immediately. In case of doubt second look laparotomy can be done 24 to 48 hours later.

Acute thrombotic occlusion produces much more extensive bowel ischemia due to diffuse nature of the disease. Usually CA and SMA both are involved in the process. Hence aorta to CA-SMA bypass is usually required. If bowel resection is required great saphenous vein is the preferred conduit for bypass which is infection resistant. Otherwise Dacron/PTFE graft, either bifurcated or sequential, can be used in antegrade manner. Sometimes retrograde bypass from infrarenal aorta or common iliac artery to SMA/CA is done due to emergency situation to cut short ischemia time and operating time. Supraceliac aortic dissection and control is a time consuming procedure. Also in severe cardiac disease patient may not tolerate clamping of supraceliac aorta. But retrograde graft is more prone for kinking after bowel is restored to abdomen.

Chronic mesenteric ischemia—If thrombotic occlusion of SMA and CA is near the orifice, transaortic endarterectomy can be performed. For more than 2 cm distal lesions bypass graft is required as described earlier (Figs 12.3 and 12.4).

In NOMI—As mentioned earlier transcatheter papaverine 30-60 mg/hour is given. Concomitantly heparin is given to prevent thrombosis in treated vessel. Systemic absorption of papaverine leads to hypotension and hence proximal catheter migration must be watched. If signs of bowel ischemia develop clinically, infusion of papaverine should be continued and abdomen explored.

Celiac artery compression—Occurs in young females between 20 and 45 years of age, presenting with upper abdominal pain precipitated by meals. With this presentation, the diagnosis should be suspected. Angiogram in lateral projection shows significant CA compression during expiration. This compression needs to be released surgically. Sometimes, CA stenosis is present which needs to be bypassed using a suitable conduit.

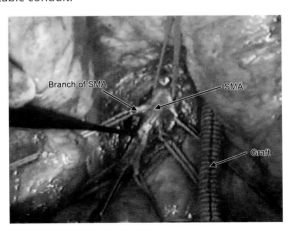

Fig. 12.3: Retrograde visceral bypass

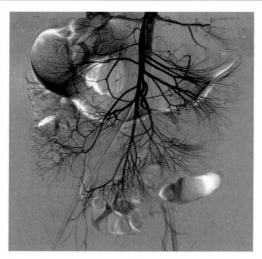

Fig. 12.4: Completion angiogram after visceral bypass

Mesenteric Vein Thrombosis

It accounts for approximately 20% cases of undiagnosed abdominal pain and is of two types:

1. *Primary MVT:* Here the cause of venous thrombosis is not obvious.
2. *Secondary MVT:* This could be due to variety of causes as follows:
   - Liver cirrhosis
   - Splenic vein thrombosis after splenectomy
   - Hypercoagulable state due to deficiency of protein C, S, and AT III, APC resistance, anticardiolipin antibodies syndrome, malignancy, polycythemia vera, etc.
   - Intra-abdominal infection following appendicular perforation causing portal pyemia.
   - May follow sclerotherapy for esophageal varices, transhepatic portal angiography, liver transplant, TIPS, etc.

Clinical Features

Patient may be asymptomatic or may present with prolonged abdominal discomfort. There could be signs of peritonitis if bowel injury is associated with venous thrombosis. Abdomen may be distended due to bowel edema, fluid and bloody diarrhea may occur due to bowel infarction, which is a bad prognostic sign. Some patients have ascites. Isolated splenic vein thrombosis does not produce bowel ischemia but produces signs of portal hypertension.

Treatment

It mainly consists of systemic anticoagulation with unfractionated heparin or LMWH followed by oral anticoagulant for adequate length of time. Catheter directed thrombolysis is possible in acute cases detected in time. Resolution of thrombus may be monitored with duplex ultrasound and also assessed by clinical improvement.

Conduits in Vascular Surgery

Conduits are required in vascular surgery to establish the blood flow beyond obstruction or to bridge the gap between two segments of vessels. Various types of vascular conduits are available presently, but the search for 'ideal conduit' is never ending process. Following features are expected of an ideal conduit:

1. Readily available off the shelf.
2. Should be available in all sizes.
3. Should be easy to handle, i.e. should be elastic and compliant.
4. Cut ends should not fray and conduit should not kink at joints.
5. Should be resistant to infection.
6. Should be least thrombogenic.
7. Should be durable, nontoxic and nonallergic to body tissues.
8. Should be biostable and nonimmunogenic.

In short, it should be similar in characters to artery or vein it is replacing. Only autogenous arterial conduits fulfill all the criteria.

Vascular conduits/grafts are of mainly two types:
1. Biological grafts: These are of three types:
    *   Autogenous grafts
    *   Allografts
    *   Xenografts
2. Prosthetic grafts.

Autogenous Grafts (Figs 13.1 and 13.2)

These are harvested from patient's own body and can be arterial or venous grafts.

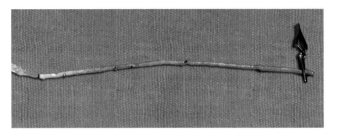

Fig. 13.1: Great saphenous vein harvested

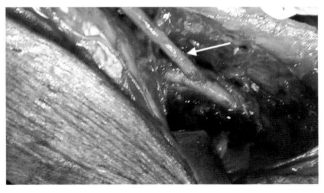

Fig. 13.2: Pta—reversed saphenous vein graft

Arterial grafts: Various arterial grafts available are radial artery, inferior hypogastric artery and thrombosed (superficial) femoral artery after cleaning the thrombus.

Advantages

- Potential for growth when used in children
- Nonthrombogenic
- Compliant, easy to suture, least kinking
- Resistant to infection hence can be used in infected/contaminated area for primary anastomosis/reconstruction, to replace infected prosthetic graft or anastomotic false aneurysm.

Disadvantages

Small sized arteries like internal thoracic artery is reserved for coronary artery bypass grafting. Radial artery is also frequently used for CABG surgery. Hence only limited arterial conduits are available for vascular anastomosis. Size and length of the available conduit also needs consideration before use. Hence arterial conduits though ideal are very scanty. Thrombosed SFA if excised can be cleaned of thrombus and may be suitable in selected situations.

Autogenous Vein

Various autogenous venous conduits available are great saphenous vein (GSV), small saphenous vein, cephalic and basilic veins. Rarely iliac and femoral veins have been considered for interposition for large size arterial revascularization if venous drainage is not hampered. By far the most commonly used conduit is great saphenous vein which is suitable for small and medium size arterial revascularization.

Advantages

- Readily available on most of the occasions.
- Adequate length and caliber vein usually available.
- Easy to handle and suture, can be used as a patch also.
- Resistant to infection.
- Biocompatible, flexible. Kink resistant even at joints.
- If handled carefully, it is minimally thrombogenic.

Disadvantages

- Nonavailability of autogenous vein due to varicosity, previously used for CABG surgery, or thrombosed vein or damaged due to trauma. This can occur in 10-20% cases.
- Sometimes, the size of the vein is small and vein smaller than 2.5 mm is not suitable for vascular anastomosis. Thus size mismatch is a definite disadvantage. Also GSV is not suitable for suprapopliteal bypass.
- Harvesting vein is a time consuming procedure and produces morbidity >20% due to long incision. If it is harvested through small incisions, excessive pulling and stretching it produces definite intimal damage and compromises long- term patency.
- In obese patients with bulky thighs, sometimes, it is difficult to locate GSV and more dissection and time may be required.
- The GSV is to be reversed for anastomosis to orient the valves direction of blood flow. In this process, distal smaller end of the reversed vein goes to proximal end of the artery which is larger, producing size mismatch. Also excision from the bed damages vasa vasorum jeopardizing the blood supply to the vein wall. These problems can be obviated by using GSV *in situ* and intraluminal valves are to be resected by valvulotome or under angioscopic guidance.
- Placed in the arterial circulation, intimal hyperplasia occurs producing narrowing of graft lumen. Average patency rate is 50% at 5 years.

Allografts

Modified human umbilical vein (HUV) graft: Nowadays, HUV is procured by computer controlled process and tanned with glutaraldehyde. The later produces collagen conduit devoid of endothelium. It eliminates immunogenic reaction but increases thrombogenicity due to lack of endothelium.

Advantages

The HUV graft is useful in limb-threatening ischemia, in the presence of infection and tissue loss. It is available off the shelf and is a good alternative when other grafts are not available. Cryogenically preserved grafts have improved performance.

Disadvantages

- Special procedure is required for procurement and preservation of HUV. Before finally implanting it special washing technique is to be followed.
- Biodegradation and aneurysm formation are common.
- Delicate handling is required. Pulling through tunnel damages the graft. Hence, it is to be protected by metal sheath and then negotiated. It must be mentioned here that the enthusiasm to use HUV graft is not great.

Prosthetic Grafts

Dacron Grafts

It was first patented as Dacron in 1950. It is made up of polyethylene terephthalate and is available in two forms.
i. Knitted Dacron
ii. Woven Dacron

Knitted Dacron (Fig. 13.3)

Dacron threads are looped to form continuous interlocking chain mostly in longitudinal pattern. This gives good porosity

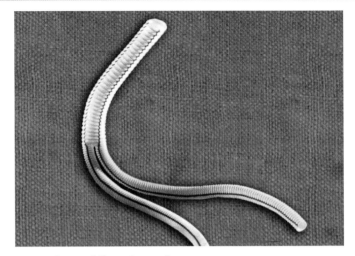

Fig. 13.3: Dacron bifurcation graft

with radial distensibility. Handling is better. But due to porosity bleeding through holes is more, which may become significant sometimes. Hence preclotting is must in knitted graft. It is less strong and subject to more structural, changes and dilatation in due course.

Coated Dacron grafts: Coating with gelatin, collagen or albumin has been provided which seals the pores. Hence preclotting is not required. The reagents are degraded in the body from 2 weeks (gelatin, collagen) to 2 months (albumin). After implantation fibrin, platelets, blood cells, foreign body giant cells get deposited on inner aspect and connective tissue is deposited on the outer aspect from few hours to few months. Middle layer remains acellular.

Dacron double velour grafts: Dacron graft can be modified by extending loops of yarn on both internal and external surfaces by velour technique. Due to external velour graft is firmly incorporated into surrounding tissues, while internally it may enhance firm anchorage of fibrin/platelet pseudointima. Velour adds to elasticity and decreases porosity.

Heparin bonding has been provided in some grafts to decrease thrombogenicity, but whether it is really helpful remains to be proved.

Woven Dacron

Here Dacron threads are fabricated by over and under pattern. Hence, the porosity is limited. Consequently, bleeding through the graft is less and structural deformation is less likely. Disadvantages are reduced compliance and less desirable handling. There is reduced tissue incorporation and cut edges tend to fray, hence less suitable for suturing.

Expanded Polymer of Polytetrafluoroethylene Grafts (Figs 13.4 to 13.7)

It is an expanded polymer of polytetrafluoroethylene (ePTFE), originally patented as 'Teflon' in 1937 by Dupont. In this graft fine fibrils extend between solid nodes, the distance between nodes being 30 microns. There is less biological degradation. Surface of the graft is electronegative; hence there is less reaction with blood components. Carbon coating has been used in newer grafts to increase electronegativity and thus to reduce chances of thrombus formation. Thin-walled grafts (0.2-0.3 mm) are available for better compliance and handling. Stretch grafts are available where due to stretching length can be increased as per requirement. Addition of rings or coils on the outer surface prevents collapse of the graft, prevents kinking near joint lines and also takes care of extrinsic compression. Patency of ePTFE graft in above knee position is excellent, but in below knee position it is inferior to reversed GSV graft. Hence for infrapopliteal bypasses, it is not a preferred

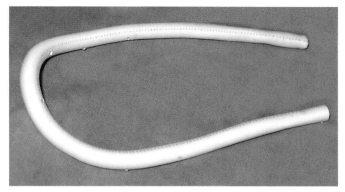

Fig. 13.4: PTFE graft

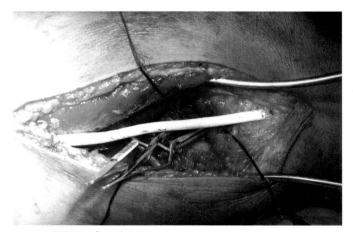

Fig. 13.5: PTFE graft to CFA

conduit. Some modifications have been carried out at distal end like precuffed design to increase patency in below knee position. Vein cuff modification has shown better efficacy in

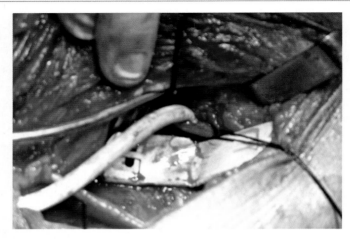

Fig. 13.6: PTFE graft end-side to CFA

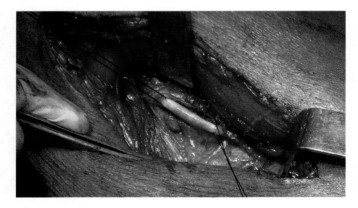

Fig. 13.7: PTFE interposition graft

infrapopliteal application and for dialysis angioaccess. Silver impregnated grafts have become available recently, which are supposed to offer resistance to infection.

The ePTFE grafts are the most commonly used conduits these days due to easy availability in various sizes suitable for small diameter vessel of 3 mm to large vessel like aorta. Bifurcation graft, grafts with side arms, etc. are available. Various features mentioned above make them useful conduits for routine use, except for the cost.

Polyurethane Graft

It was used initially in left ventricular assist device, coating for artificial heart, in implantable roller pumps. The material is compliant, elastic and biocompatible. Small size grafts like ones suitable for coronary artery bypass surgery, for dialysis angioaccess are made up of polyurethane. So far its superiority over Dacron or ePTFE grafts has not been proved by authentic studies. Pseudointimal proliferation at the end of the graft is more and carcinogenic effect of products of degradation of polyurethane is the matter of real concern presently. But it appears to be a promising material for the future.

Hence vascular surgeon has opportunity to choose conduit depending on the patient's economic status, emergency or planned situation, presence of infection or otherwise, general condition of the patient, etc. Even joint grafts called 'composite graft' can be used, for example, femoral artery to posterior tibial artery bypass where above knee segment is replaced with ePTFE and below knee with reversed great saphenous vein and both grafts are joined in the middle. Prosthetic grafts of frequently used sizes should always be kept ready off the shelf in a vascular center to avoid eleventh hour rush for the graft.

Endovascular Interventions

Modern vascular surgeon must be well-versed with the endovascular technique because he has to perform the task of a physician, a surgeon as well as of an interventional specialist, as dependence on cardiologist and interventional radiologist takes away major vascular work. Many vascular surgeons have general knowledge about endovascular interventions but firsthand experience of performing these procedures is usually lacking. This chapter gives basic information about endovascular procedures under following heads:

   i. Vascular access
  ii. Maintaining vascular access
 iii. Endovascular devices
- Guidewires
- Catheters
  - Diagnostic catheters
  - Guiding catheters
  - Balloon angioplasty catheters
- Intravascular stents
- Atherectomy
  iv. Technique
   v. Results.

Vascular Access

To start with one has to gain access to the lumen of the vessel which is commonly performed by percutaneous puncture of the vessel. Occasionally, direct access to the vessel may be required surgically due to difficulty in percutaneous access. The optimal puncture site should be near to the target vessel of intervention; site should have low rate of complications and should be easy to convert into open surgery if required. Compression should be possible to stop bleed after the procedure. *Common femoral artery is thus the best site for access (and common femoral vein for venous access).* Three types of needles are available for percutaneous access.

Single Wall Puncture Needle

It is most commonly used in the size of 16-18G, which has hollow needle with guidewire 0.035". After locating the artery by palpation and keeping two fingers apart along its length the needle is inserted at 45 degree angle to the skin and pushed to enter the lumen of the artery which is confirmed by free, pulsatile flow of red blood. Then guidewire is advanced.

Double Wall Puncture Needle

It has two components, i.e. outer hollow needle which has blunt tip and the inner bevel tipped stylet which just projects out of the tip of needle. Whole assembly is pushed at 45 degree angle till it hits the bone. Then stylet is removed and needle is gradually withdrawn till good free blood flow is obtained. Due to additional puncture of the posterior wall of the vessel this technique may produce more bleeding complications.

Micropuncture Needle

It is a variation of single needle technique wherein 21G puncture needle is used and 0.018" nitinol guidewire is advanced. This has less bleeding complications.

Smart Needle Technique

It is used when target vessel is pulse less and located near important structures. It is 16G needle with inner stylet has 14 MHz Doppler transducer probe for localizing the best signal for puncture.

Technique of Vascular Access

Retrograde puncture of CFA is the most commonly performed technique, because of the large size of the artery and as it can be compressed against femoral head. The needle is advanced through skin at 45 degree angle into CFA till good pulsatile flow is obtained. Though it is usually a safe approach, complications can occur due to improper technique as follows:

a. Puncture above inguinal ligament can produce retroperitoneal hematoma.

b. Proximal puncture of femoral artery can produce thrombosis.

c. Proximal profunda femoris artery puncture is difficult to compress and hence can produce hemorrhage.

- Antegrade CFA puncture is actually a difficult approach due to body contours and limited working space available between puncture site and CFA bifurcation. Placing folded towel beneath the hip and retracting the lower abdomen upwards abdomen by assistant or by taping it greatly help for antegrade puncture. It is helpful to study ipsilateral distal vascular system.

- *Retrograde popliteal artery puncture:* When CFA puncture is not possible due to groin problem popliteal artery can be punctured in prone position under USG guidance. Similarly, axillary and brachial arteries can be punctured if bilateral CFA are nonpulsatile.

- Venous cannulation is required frequently, e.g. internal jugular vein cannulation for RA/SVC pressure monitoring and for drugs say for example for open heart surgery; CFV cannulation for thrombolysis and intervention, etc.

Maintaining Vascular Access

After gaining vascular access, it needs to be maintained so that repeated puncture is not required. The access is maintained by guidewire. For diagnostic procedure, full length guidewire is inserted and diagnostic catheter is advanced over it into the vessel to be studied. Flush aortography (or vena cavography) can be performed with this technique. For any other intervention for selective catheterization use of introducer sheath is a must. The most commonly used sheath is 5-6 F size (1F=0.033 mm or 0.013"). Larger sheath is required for deploying stents, stent grafts, devices, etc. Sheath has two ports—one for the guidewire and side port for pressure monitoring, blood sampling and for drugs. Due to hemostatic valve back bleed from the sheath valve is prevented. Exchange of guidewires, diagnostic catheters, interventional catheters and devices all are performed through the lumen of the sheath thus reducing the likely injury to the vessel wall due to their repeated passage. Sheaths are available in various lengths. 10-12 cm is the standard length in majority of the peripheral vascular procedures.

Endovascular Devices

Guidewires

Function of the angiographic guidewires is to facilitate position of the catheter in particular location by supporting and guiding the same. It has two components: (a) Inner wire is called 'mandrel' which tapers towards the tip to produce floppy tip and (b) Outer component is stainless steel wrap, the tip of which is connected to the tip of mandrel for safety. But in movable core wire the mandrel can be moved inside. In infusion guidewire inner core wire can be removed and infusion given through outer channel. Terumo guidewire has mandrel made of nitinol and outer core of polyurethane and is very slippery.

The tip of the guidewire could be J tip, straight or angled. J tip is least traumatic, least likely to dissect but least likely to negotiate a tight stenosis. Most commonly J tip has 1.5-3 mm radius and standard length is 145-180 cm, which is useful for catheter positioning and for catheter exchange length required is 240-300 cm.

The diameter is variable but usual diameter is 0.035" (range 0.012-0.052"). Newer wires are coming with balloon at the tip to prevent distal embolization, e.g. in carotid stenting and in coronary artery interventions.

Catheters

Diagnostic Catheters

These are meant to deliver contrast material into the vascular system to opacify the flow channel of the vessel under study. These are of two types:

i. Nonselective diagnostic catheters which are the ones used for study of aorta and IVC (Figs 14.1 A to C).

ii. Selective catheters are designed to engage in the orifice of branch vessel and by contrast injection selective opacification of vessel under study is carried out, e.g. renal, superior mesenteric arteries, etc. Catheter tip shape (premade or manual), stiffness, response to torque (rotation from outside), radiopacity, whether side holes are present at the tip, etc. are among the various features which decide their use. Usual length is 65-100 cm which depends on

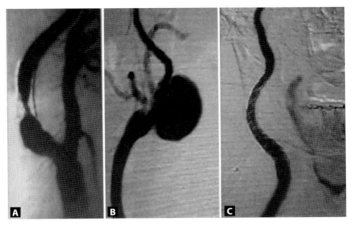

Figs 14.1A to C: Aortogram showing aneurysm

which location it is going to be used. Diagnostic catheters typically used for peripheral work is of 4-6 F size and having internal diameter ID of 0.035-0.038"usually.

Following diagnostic catheters are generally used:

a. Straight tip catheter for general arteriography
b. Bernstein catheter (self-forming) for general arteriography
c. Cobra catheter (self-forming) for branch and contralateral iliac
d. Tennis racket catheter for aortography
e. Simmons (manual forming) for contralateral iliac, subclavian, carotid
f. Shepherd Hook (manual) for renal, mesenteric, aortic bifurcation crossing

Other uses of diagnostic catheters are:

- To instil pharmacological agents (Fig. 14.2)
- Delivery of embolic material
- Sampling of blood from specific areas
- Pressure measurement.

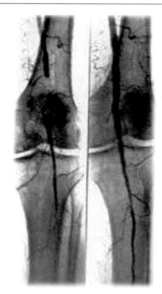

Fig. 14.2: Popliteal artery thrombolysis

Guiding Catheters

These are large diameter catheters which require larger puncture. They are usually preshaped to self-forming curves and allow the passage of balloon catheter and interventional devices. Due to their large size they allow injection of contrast medium with the presence of balloon catheter and guidewire inside. Guiding catheter also helps to determine appropriate positioning of balloon catheter or stent prior to its inflation or deployment. It also provides external support to the device due to its stiffness. These are helpful in performing angioplasty of distant, contralateral site and also used for passage of snares, graspers to protect the wall of the vessel. Typical sizes used are 6-10 F outer diameter OD.

Balloon Angioplasty Catheters

Present day balloons are made up of polyethylene, polyester and woven Dacron for peripheral angioplasty. Maximum inflation pressure of the balloon differs from balloon to balloon ranging from 12 atm to 17 atm. Balloon diameter ranges from 1.5 mm to 18 mm, up to 5 mm in the increments of 0.5 mm and above 5 mm in the increments of 1 mm. Ideally the balloon diameter should be 10-20% greater than the diameter of the adjacent normal vessel. Balloon catheters are available in 40, 75, and 120 cm usable lengths. Adequate length catheter to reach from vascular access site to the lesion in the vessel to be treated is selected. Balloon length is usually 2.0, 4.0 and 10 cm. Around less than 30% residual stenosis after balloon angioplasty indicates a good result.

Cutting balloons introduced for coronary stenosis are useful for angioplasty of small arteries like tibial and renal artery branch stenosis, which are not suitable for stenting. High pressure balloon resistant stenosis or in-stent restenosis can be treated with cutting balloon. It should be of the size of the vessel and not oversize and should not be used in totally occluded or tortuous vessel. Balloon is slowly inflated and blades expand radially into the lesion making grooves in plaque. The lesion may become suitable for stenting sometimes.

Intravascular Stents (Figs 14.3 and 14.4)

Stents are the devices which are deployed to compress, dilate the intravascular obstruction and to maintain it to avoid collapse again. They can be classified based on various features but most commonly on the basis of their method of deployment. Thus, there are two basic types:

I. Balloon expanded stent
II. Self-expanding stent

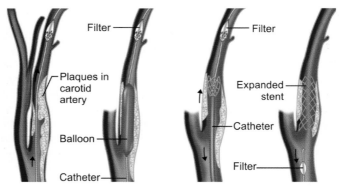

Fig. 14.3: Carotid artery stenting

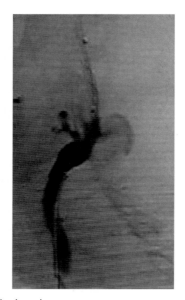

Fig. 14.4: Stent deployed

Balloon Expanded Stent

Presently fifth generation of balloon expandable stents are available. Most common type used is Palmaz stent. After deployment the stent is inflated with balloon. If required further balloon dilation is possible to increase its diameter further, this is required sometimes to avoid dislodgement. To avoid dislodgement of the stent while negotiating tortuous vessel, it is best passed through sheath or guiding catheter. Once in position across the lesion, sheath or guiding catheter is retracted and balloon is inflated at required pressure deploying the stent.

Self-expanding Stent

It is oversized to fit in the vessel without dislodgement. After retracting the delivery system the stent expands spontaneously. It cannot be dilated further by balloon. Hence proper size selection is very important. Self-expanding stents are flexible, conformable to the tortuosity of the vessel. Although they are advanced through vascular system without sheath or guiding catheter, they are encased by outer sheath which comes as part of the delivery system and it maintains the stent in collapsed state. Once in position, the outer catheter is retracted and the stent is deployed. Commonly used self-expanding stents are— Nitinol symphony, stainless steel and Wall stent.

Drug eluting stents coated with sirolimus or paclitaxel are latest addition to this group which due to slow release of drugs overcomes the problem of restenosis. These are being commonly used in coronary stenosis.

Stents covered with Dacron or ePTFE are presently available for treatment of aneurysms, pseudoaneurysms, arteriovenous fistula, arterial perforation, etc. Endovascular repair of abdominal and thoracic aortic aneurysm (EVAR) is the latest and challenging development in this category.

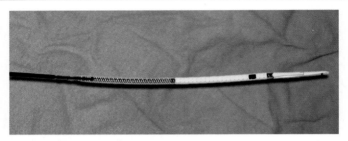

Fig. 14.5: Atherectomy device

Complications of stent:
- *Acute*: Dissection, occlusion, arterial rupture, migration or embolization of stent, embolism of atherosclerotic material
- *Chronic*: Intimal hyperplasia, recurrent stenosis, infection and stent damage.

Atherectomy: It is a procedure by which atherosclerotic plaque burden can be reduced to establish blood flow distally (Fig. 14.5). It is advocated when balloon angioplasty is not possible due to hard plaque. It can be done either by percutaneous route or though small arteriotomy. Two types of devices are available:
I.   This type removes obstruction by cutting or shaving the atheroma and debris is removed in collecting chamber, e.g. Simpson's atherotrack.
II. Ablative atherectomy device has a high speed rotational head to pulverize the plaque to smaller fragments that can be aspirated mechanically or removed through reticuloendothelial system of the host.

Results

Are inferior to conventional bypass and there is a high restenosis rate due to intimal hyperplasia. It is a tedious and time consuming procedure and is useful only for short segment lesion. Complications like bleeding, hematoma, thrombosis, arterial rupture, embolization, catheter fracture, death are likely to occur.

Technique

Details of technique like gaining access, maintaining it, use of guidewire, catheters, etc. have been described under various heads and need not to be repeated.

Results

Can be assessed in three ways:

I. By using intravascular ultrasound (IVUS) postprocedure assessment of successful opening of obstructing lesion is best done. But as this modality is not available to majority of the centers, it cannot be quoted as routine assessment measure.

II. Postprocedure completion angiography is the best available technique as the gadgets are still inside and doing angiography is easy. But the presence of guidewire, catheter, etc. distort the image and artefacts may interfere with proper assessment and it may not be possible to inject sufficient contrast medium. Still majority of the angioplasties and stents performed are assessed with completion angiography only. Dissection which does not extend beyond the dilated area and does not obstruct the flow should be viewed as successful outcome. On the contrary satisfactory angiographic result may be hemodynamically suboptimal owing to the limitations of angiography. As written earlier <30% residual stenosis is considered successful result of the procedure.

III. Pressure measurement proximal and distal to the treated lesion may give clue to the result. Pressure drop of 5-10 mm Hg is considered normal and pressure difference of > 20 mm Hg is significant and heralds future restenosis.

Follow-up of the patients is done 1, 3 and 6 months after the procedure with duplex ultrasound. Greater than 50% stenosis on DUS is considered clinically significant for which further intervention is to be considered.

Chronic Venous Insufficiency

Venous Anatomy

Chronic venous insufficiency (CVI) is a serious socioeconomic problem affecting 1-2% of population and above the age of 65 years more than 4% population may be affected. All of them without exception experience physical incapacity leading to diminution of work capacity which leads to loss of more than 2 million working days every year and billions of rupees.

Etiology

There are three important causes for CVI:
1. Varicose veins
2. Deep vein thrombosis sequelae
3. Incompetent perforator veins

Note: Refer to the Chapter 16 on varicose veins and deep vein thrombosis.

Pathophysiology

Veins are distensible, thin-walled structures which carry the blood from periphery, i.e. from limbs towards heart which is aided by muscular contractions of calf muscles hence called "peripheral heart". Regurgitation of blood is avoided by unidirectional valves present in the veins. These intraluminal valves may become incompetent due to varicose veins or due to destruction in previous deep vein thrombosis causing fibrosis and distortion. This leads to reflux of blood on standing erect by gravity or hydrostatic pressure leading to ambulatory venous hypertension. Calf muscles produce 150-300 mm Hg intracompartmental pressure (hydrodynamic pressure) during muscular contraction which pushes blood towards heart through deep veins. In case of perforator vein reflux the hydrodynamic pressure pushes blood from deep veins to superficial veins due to incompetent valves which in addition to hydrostatic pressure, increase ambulatory venous pressure tremendously, which is the important cause of CVI sequelae. In addition to this cause for reflux, obstruction in deep veins due to persistent or partly recanalized DVT adds to venous hypertension. Thus, reflux or combined reflux and obstruction in combination cause CVI. Role of isolated perforator vein incompetence is debatable.

When the cause for valvular reflux is not clear, it is called *Primary CVI* and if the cause of valvular reflux is obvious mostly being secondary to DVT, it is called *Secondary CVI*.

Numerous theories were proposed earlier concerning etiology and pathophysiology of CVI. Theories like venous stasis, AV fistula and diffusion block theories have been found to be irrelevant.

Leukocyte Activation Theory

Due to venous hypertension, neutrophils are trapped in microcirculation and capillary blood flow becomes sluggish leading to hypoxia of tissues. This leads to neutrophil activation and degradation of tissue metabolites causing endothelial damage, which in turn leads to altered skin blood flow. Consequently, lysozomal enzymes are released and skin damage is produced producing clinical picture of CVI.

Secondary to venous hypertension, extravasation of macro-molecules like fibrinogen, alpha-2 macroglobulin and red blood cells occurs in dermal interstitium which produces chronic inflammatory response which is responsible for stasis derma-titis. TGF-B1 appears to be a primary regulator of CVI induced injury.

Clinical Features

Based on the theories mentioned above clinical features can be explained. Majority complain of leg fatigue, aching, night cramps, discomfort and heaviness in legs. They may present with leg edema which is initially pitting and later on becomes less so due to chronicity. Varicose veins are present in many which could be either primary or secondary. Skin hyperpigmentation, lipodermatosclerosis and in extreme cases venous ulcers may occur (Figs 15.1 and 15.2). Venous ulcers are located on medial side of leg related to medial malleolus, which do not heal over

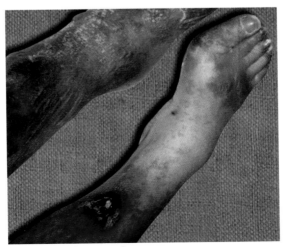

Fig. 15.1: Post-thrombotic syndrome

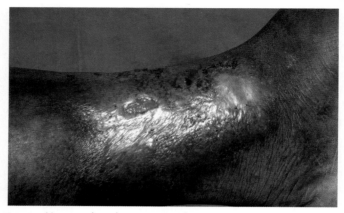

Fig. 15.2: Venous ulcer due to venous hypertension

a prolonged period of time and may occur even without clinical evidence of any varicosity.

Clinical Classification

Clinical signs, etiology, anatomical distribution and pathophysiological dysfunction (CEAP) classification was conceptualized in 1994 by International Consensus Committee meeting sponsored by American Venous Forum and is being used world over for reporting on venous disorders for uniformity. The details of the same are as follows:

C—Clinical signs A—Asymptomatic S—Symptomatic

Class 0: No visible/palpable signs of venous disease

Class 1: Telangiectasia, reticular veins, malleolar flush

Class 2: Varicose veins

Class 3: Edema, no skin changes

Class 4: Skin changes, e.g. hyperpigmentation, lipodermatosclerosis, and eczema.

Class 5: Skin changes + healed ulcer
Class 6: Skin changes + active ulcer.

E—Etiology

Congenital (Ec): Venous disorder present from birth
Primary (Ep): Chronic venous disorder of unknown cause
Secondary (Es): Venous disorder secondary to, e.g. post-thrombotic, posttraumatic cause.

A—Anatomical distribution

A s_{1-5}: Superficial veins
A $_{D6-16}$: Deep veins
A_{P17-18}: Perforating veins.

P—Pathophysiological dysfunction

P_R: Reflux
P_O: Obstruction
P_{RO}: Reflux and obstruction.

The CEAP classification is very helpful in describing the venous disorder and planning the management.

Differential Diagnosis

Polyarteritis nodosa, acanthosis, lymphedema, Marjolin's ulcer Idiopathic cramps and fungal infections.

Investigations

Duplex ultrasound (DUS) is a combination of real time B mode with Doppler ultrasound. Addition of color flow signals makes it triplex ultrasound scanning, which is an excellent, most commonly used modality to evaluate CVI subjects. It identifies involved segment of venous tree and reflux lasting more than 0.5 seconds when cuff pressure is released. Persistent thrombus or partly resolved thrombus in deep veins with destruction of valves can be diagnosed. Only difficulty is in imaging veins above inguinal ligaments and in the vicinity of metallic prosthesis inserted for orthopedic injuries.

Invasive investigations are rarely advised in the following situations:

A. When clinical examination and DUS are insufficient to provide complete diagnosis
B. When endovascular intervention or deep vein surgery is planned.

Venography: It is done by injecting radiopaque dye in dorsal arch vein of foot and the passage upwards is studied. This is called ascending Venography which is important for the diagnosis of deep vein obstruction. It can also be used as access for thrombolysis, for balloon dilatation of stenosis and for inserting stent. Descending Venography is done through proximal puncture and it is important to assess reflux across deep venous valves which are important for planning reconstruction.

Magnetic Resonance Venography is also becoming popular technique for the same purpose and is noninvasive. It is better for venous study than for arterial disease evaluation.

Ambulatory venous pressure (AVP) along with Venous Recovery Time (VRT):

The AVP is recorded by the venipuncture of the dorsal arch vein which is connected to pressure transducer. Patient is asked to perform 10 tip-toe exercises. Gradually the pressure recorded by transducer stabilizes and reflects a balance between venous inflow and outflow. This is an AVP. Exercise is stopped and the vein is allowed to fill. The pressure is allowed to recover to baseline. Time required to reach 90% of the AVP is called VRT. Increased AVP indicates venous hypertension and its magnitude the severity of CVI. With AVP of 80 mm Hg or more, there is >80% incidence of developing CVI and ulceration.

Plethysmography: It measures volume changes in calf with positional changes and after tip-toe exercises. Infrared light is used in venous photoplethysmography (PPG) placed just above medial malleolus and patient then performs tip-toe exercises. It does not give accurate AVP but provides adequate VRT measurement, which is shortened in CVI. But it does not give localization. During air plethysmography (APG) air filled bladder is used around calf to measure volume changes in calf in different positions.

Intravascular ultrasound (IVUS) is a new modality, which is useful to directly visualize the interior of the veins, hence nature of intraluminal valves, thrombosis can be seen. It is especially, useful to study intra-abdominal venous compression and is more sensitive than venography and pressure studies.

Management of Chronic Venous Insufficiency

Nonoperative management is the mainstay of CVI treatment, which includes compression therapy, skin substitutes and drug therapy as described below:

Compression Therapy (Fig. 15.3)

The mechanism by which this helps is not clearly understood. Some have found changes in AVP and VRT with compression whereas other groups have not noted any difference. It may cause increase in subcutaneous interstitial pressure, which counteracts transcapillary leakage/diffusion. Thus, it could result in better fluid resorption, decrease in edema, and better diffusion of nutrients to skin and subcutaneous tissues. Increase in skin $tcPO_2$ has therefore been observed by many indicating better perfusion. Compression can be carried out in following ways:

a. Elastic compression stockings with pressure of 30-40 mm Hg at ankle are usually prescribed for established CVI with ulcer. Stockings are pulled on limb in lying down position to reduce AVP and then the patient has to get up. It must be worn throughout the day, i.e. during erect posture and

STYLE

| A-D calf | A-G thigh | A-G thigh with waist attachment |

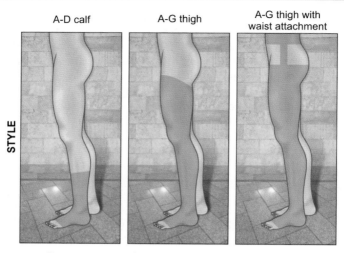

Fig. 15.3: Compression stockings

can be removed during night, when the limb is to be kept elevated on folded mattress supporting complete limb. If such elevation causes backache, it can be avoided, but then stockings should be worn even during night. In case painful ulcer is not allowing tight compression, initially light pressure garments should be tried. Skin colored stockings are available for better cosmesis. Multilayered compression bandage technique has been used for CVI with ulcer on indoor basis, the compression being maintained constantly with better ulcer healing.

Ninety-three percent persons who were compliant had complete ulcer healing within 5 months. Recurrence rate was 16%, but it was 100% in noncompliant patients. The recurrence was not related to previous ulcer, previous venous surgery or arterial insufficiency.

b. *Unna boot:* Paul Gerson Unna, a German dermatogist developed this boot in 1896. It consists of three layered dressing to be applied by trained person. A roller gauge bandage impregnated with calamine, zinc oxide, glycerin, sorbitol, gelatine and magnesium alum silicate is first applied with graded compression from forefoot to below knee level. The next layer consists of 4 inch wide continuous gauge dressing followed by elastic wrap outer layer. The bandage becomes stiff after drying which helps to reduce edema. It is changed weekly. Ulcer healing to the extent of 73% has been observed in 9 weeks.

   Disadvantages: It is uncomfortable for the patient, ulcer healing cannot be monitored, and compression applied is operator dependent. More fluid discharge cannot be taken care of and contact dermatitis may occur.

c. *Intermittent pneumatic compression (IPC):* This can be used on outpatient basis. Using pressure cuffs at multiple levels sequential compression is given from periphery towards heart. Level of pressure can be selected. For compliant patients willing to take long-term therapy it is a good option.

Contraindications for compression therapy:

i. Peripheral arterial disease
ii. Cellulitis, infected painful ulcers, which should be treated with antibiotics, analgesics and dressings before starting compression therapy.

Skin Substitutes

Apligraf is a commercially available living skin substitute, which closely matches human skin. It is between 0.5 and 1 mm thick and is applied as a disk of living tissue on an agarose gel nutrient medium. Sixty-three percent ulcers healed within 60 days, which is better than compression therapy alone.

Pharmacological Therapy

Various drugs have been tried to treat CVI.

i. *Phlebotrophic drugs:* Hydroxyrutosides, flavonoids derived from plants glycosides showed improvement in pain, restless legs and nocturnal cramps but no difference has been observed in ulcer healing.

Micronized purified flavonoids fraction (MPFF) is a combination of micronized flavonoids and diosmin with marginal improvement in CVI status.

Calcium dobesilate reduces edema by increasing lymphatic flow and macrophage mediated proteolysis. Symptoms of CVI showed improvement on this drug.

Troxerutin has antierythrocyte effect and may improve capillary dynamics in patients with mild CVI. Effect on ulcer healing is unknown.

ii. Pentoxifylline is a hemorheological agent, which reduces neutrophil adhesiveness, inhibits cytokine mediated neutrophil activation and reduces the release superoxide free radicals produced in neutrophil degradation. Better ulcer healing has been reported in this group.

iii. Prostaglandin E1 reduces WBC activation, inhibits platelet aggregation and decreases small vessel dilatation. Used by intravenous route over longer period (weeks) it produces good ulcer healing (46% vs. 9%).

Interventions and Surgery for CVI and Ulcers

Patients with CVI and ulcers are treated with graded compression, Phlebotrophic drugs for minimum period of 3-6 months. If residual disease is present at the end of conservative treatment and if the disease is found to be suitable on DUS and venography, appropriate intervention is planned.

Varicose Veins

Refer to the Chapter 16 on varicose veins.

Perforator Vein Surgery

Sometimes incompetent perforator connecting superficial and deep venous systems could be the cause for localized ulcer. Linton in 1938, first ligated such perforator. This procedure is rarely used these days due to high incidence of local wound complications. Subfascial endoscopic perforator vein surgery (SEPVS), which is an endoscopic procedure done from a distant keyhole avoids direct incision in the ulcer area. This has given better result and rare wound complications as the infected area is not used for approaching and ligating perforator. Postoperative compression is maintained for 5 days and further continued for 3 weeks. Eighty-eight percent of the ulcers healed in 1 year as per the report published in North American Registry.

Venous Reconstruction

There are various techniques for doing venous reconstruction.

- *Valvuloplasty:* It is a technique employed when the valve architecture is normal, in which commissural tightening is done to reduce incompetence. It can be done by two methods:
  - Internal valvuloplasty is done by venotomy and redundant valve cusps are plicated to the vein wall using 7-0 polypropylene. This has given a durable result.
  - External valvuloplasty is a technique of blind plication of valves from outside without opening the vein lumen. Result is less satisfactory. But with the recent use of angioscope the result would definitely improve.
- *Valve transplantation:* A segment from arm vein having a competent valve is harvested and is interposed in superficial femoral vein having incompetent valve using interrupted sutures to avoid stenosis. Thus reflux is avoided due to new competent valve. But long-term results are not satisfactory.

- *Valve transposition:* This technique is used when proximal groin axial vein, e.g. profunda femoris vein or great saphenous vein has competent valve. Distal incompetent SFV is transected and anastomosed to PFV or GSV distal to competent valve so as to direct blood towards heart without reflux.
- *External banding:* Dacron or PTFE sleeve is put around incompetent valve vein segment and tightened to reduce lumen and consequently the valvular reflux. The sleeve is then fixed.
- *Valve substitutes:* These are being developed like venous valve allografts, cryopreserved, glutaraldehyde preserved bovine grafts, which may become available in future.

    Presently out of all these internal valvuloplasty has documented 60-80% long-term results, but recurrence rate is high if the ulcer was present initially.

Varicose Veins

Varicose veins is common medical condition present at least in 10% of general population.

Normally the vein wall consists of three distinct muscle layers-inner longitudinal layer, outer circular layer and adventitia has loosely organized longitudinal layers. This orderly architecture is distorted and muscle layers are replaced with disorganized deposition of collagen. Elastin content becomes less. Smooth muscle cells (SMCs) are replaced by collagen.

In deep vein thrombosis activation of neutrophils and platelets leads to chain reaction producing thrombosis and inflammation. This causes vein wall fibrosis, valvular destruction and this altered architecture produces incompetence of valves and secondary varicose veins.

Anatomy

Varicose veins are dilated, tortuous visible superficial veins in lower limbs. Telangiectasia appears like bluish discolored patches which occur due to confluence of permanently dilated intradermal venules of less than 1 mm diameter. Reticular veins are permanently dilated bluish intradermal veins usually between 1 and 3 mm in diameter. About 75% patients have saphenofemoral junction (SFJ) incompetence causing great saphenous vein varicosity. Less than 10% may have isolated small saphenous popliteal junction (SPJ) incompetence. About 20% varicose veins occur due to isolated incompetence of valves in perforating veins. Overall below knee varicose veins are more common. Rather than axial GSV, branch varicosities related to posterior arch vein and Cockett's perforators are more common.

Etiology

Though the etiology of varicose veins is not clearly understood possible factors have been suggested as below:

i. *Age:* Varicosity becomes more common with advancing age and is rare in children except in congenital variety.

ii. *Gender:* It is more common in females.

iii. *Venous stasis*: This has some correlation with occurrence of varicose veins as higher incidence is found in professions involving prolonged standing. But as the varicose veins are most common just below knee and not at ankle, indicates that stasis only is not the factor. Additional factors must be operating.

iv. *Overweight:* Obesity has higher incidence of varicose veins, but not all obese patients have varicose veins.

v. *Pregnancy:* Varicose veins occur in pregnancy or are exacerbated during pregnancy. Both mechanical compression and hormonal influences probably play their roles. Seventy to eighty percent of patients develop varicose veins during the first trimester. Later in pregnancy, increase in total blood flow in iliac veins from the uterine and ovarian veins and uterine obstruction to venous flow both may play part.

vi. *Occupation:* As mentioned above occupations involving prolonged standing like traffic policemen, surgeons have been found to be more prone for developing varicose veins.

vii. *Genetics:* Has definitely been found to have association with development of varicosity. If both parents have varicose veins, the probability of the same occurring in children is very high. The cause could be underlying defect in vein wall strength and valve structure. Dominant type of inheritance has been found in 85% of such subjects.

viii. *Previous DVT:* As already described DVT causes valvular distortion and incompetence producing secondary varicose veins.

Out of all the factors mentioned above, genetics and previous DVT are having proven association, more than other factors.

Clinical Features

Many patients may be asymptomatic initially and they seek medical advice for cosmetic reason due to dilated, tortuous veins in legs, which is a feature of the disease. Usual symptoms are leg fatigue, increased on prolonged standing, pain in calf muscles, nocturnal muscle cramps. Some may have bluish discolored patches due telangiectasia or tortuous venues and at the other extreme some may present with hugely dilated tortuous venous sacs or blow outs (Figs 16.1 and 16.2). But it is important to understand that symptoms are not proportionate to the extent of visible disease. Patients with even minor reticular veins may be highly symptomatic. Prolonged stasis in due course produces edema in legs and at ankles, which is increased at the end of the day and is trivial after getting up in the morning. Hyperpigmentation at ankle and in leg, lipodermatosclerosis (induration of skin and subcutaneous tissue), atrophy of skin and eczematoid changes occur. Venous ulceration occurs in long neglected disease usually around medial malleolus. This ulcer may bleed sometimes forcing the patient to seek medical advice in emergency.

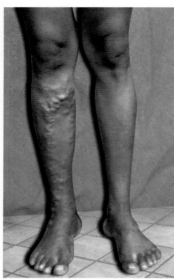

Fig. 16.1: Varicose veins

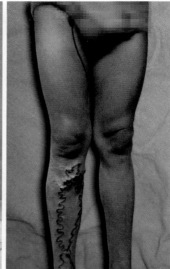

Fig. 16.2: Varicose veins marked

In congenital variety like Klippel-Trenaunay syndrome children or younger patients present with tortuous venous sacs on lateral aspect of upper thigh, while the axial veins are normal (Fig. 16.3).

Pathophysiology

Hydrostatic pressure is a gravitational force which produces reflux in superficial veins having incompetent intraluminal valves. Hydrodynamic pressure of 150-300 mm Hg is produced by calf muscle contractions to propel blood towards heart. In case of incompetent perforator valve this force directs blood from deep veins retrograde via perforators into superficial veins. This is a high pressure reflux. Thus combined hydrostatic and

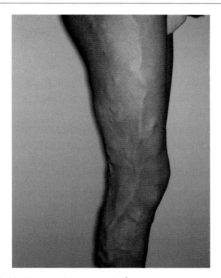

Fig. 16.3: Varicose veins—atypical

hydrodynamic pressures produce varicosities. Incompetence of the valves in communicating veins between superficial veins below superficial fascia and smaller veins in subcutaneous plane and dermis produce dilatation of reticular veins and telangiectasia. Thus venous hypertension produces venous congestion and all the related symptoms. Pressure of the dilated veins on the dense network of somatic nerves produces aching pain. Hyperpigmentation occurs due to hemosiderin deposition. If inflammatory process is triggered fibrosis occurs hardening subcutaneous tissue which is responsible for dermatosclerosis. Minor breaks in the epidermis produce ulcers which heal slowly to produce white depressed scars called "atrophie Blanche". Due to extreme rise in gravitational pressure thinned out skin on dilated varicosity may give way to produce bleeding ulcer.

Management

Medical Management

It is the initial treatment in all and the only treatment in majority of the varicose veins patients. It consists of the following:

1. Elevation of the legs during night above heart level which reduces edema and aching pain.
2. Exercises to strengthen calf muscles which avoid pulling of blood in calf venous sinuses and improves upward flow towards heart. Also leg elevation exercises in supine position have anti-gravity effect.
3. Graded compression stockings are available which give good compression over dilated veins and reduce hydrostatic pressure. These are graded depending on the compression pressure exerted at ankle level. Class I up to 18 mm Hg, Class II up to 25 mm Hg and Class III produces up to 35 mm Hg pressure at ankle. Usually for varicose veins class II stockings are adequate. But for chronic edema producing chronic venous insufficiency with ulcer class III stockings are required. They must be worn throughout the day and while wearing, the leg must be elevated to empty dilated veins. Compression stockings are advised on long-term basis if other therapy is not planned in addition.
4. Phlebotrophic drugs usually used are calcium dobesilate, micronized flavonoids and recently Troxerutin. Usually 12 weeks therapy produces good clinical result like reduction of leg edema, relief from pain in calf muscles and nocturnal cramps. Eczema and ulcers also respond to some extent. After this treatment compression stockings are continued and in selected patients further intervention is done.

Surgical Treatment (Figs 16.4 to 16.8)

Objectives

- Removal of source of hydrostatic forces by removing superficial axial vein.

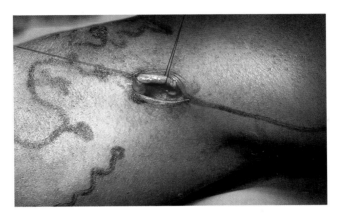

Fig. 16.4: Varicose veins—surgery dilated GSV exposed

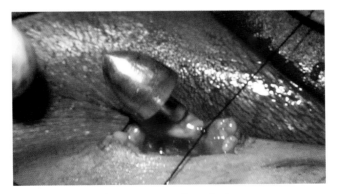

Fig. 16.5: Varicose veins—surgery stripper *in situ*

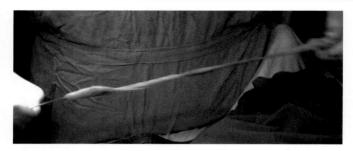

Fig. 16.6: Varicose veins—excised GSV varicosity

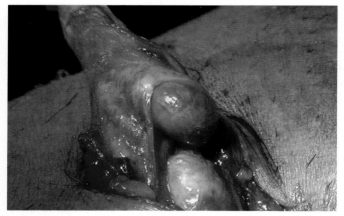

Fig. 16.7: Varicose veins—surgery venous blow out exposed

- Removal of source of hydrodynamic forces acting through perforator veins.
- Removal of additional cluster of veins for cosmesis. (All veins > 4 mm in diameter are usually removed).

Procedure: In standing position all major visible varicose veins are marked (Fig. 16.2). Under spinal anesthesia great

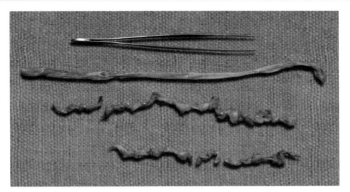

Fig. 16.8: Varicose veins—surgery excised varicose veins

saphenous vein 1 cm distal to SFJ is ligated and stripped up to few centimeter below knee. The track of stripping is compressed for few minutes to stop bleeding from avulsed perforators with thigh elevated. Below knee marked tortuous varicosities are removed by multiple stab incisions and avulsion. Bleeding is again stopped by compression. After suturing wounds compression stocking is applied and compression is maintained for about 3 weeks. Long-term results are excellent with SFJ ligation, stripping and multiple phlebectomies.

Complications: Bleeding, ecchymosis, nerve injury, lymphedema, infection and recurrence.

Sclerotherapy

Indications—ideal indications are varicose veins between 1 and 3 mm in diameter, telangiectasia, and reticular veins, isolated and below knee varicosities, residual varicose veins after surgery, recurrent varicose veins or in patients in whom surgery is risky due to advanced age or morbidity.

Patients with gross SFJ/SPJ reflux, larger varicosity > 3 mm in diameter and those with allergic reaction to sclerosant are not suitable.

Drugs used for sclerotherapy are:
- Polidocanol   Sodium tetradecyl sulfate
- Sodium morrhuate   Hypertonic saline

Injection sclerotherapy for reticular veins and telangiectasia is called microsclerotherapy and that for larger than 3 mm varicosity is called macrosclerotherapy; concentration of sclerosant for both is different.

	Microsclerotherapy	Macrosclerotherapy (Concentration)
Sclerosant		
Polidocanol	0.75%	1.0%
STD	0.25%	0.5-1%
Hypertonic saline	11.7%	23.4%

Veins are marked in standing position and punctured with 26G needle. Approximately 0.5 ml drug is injected in each varicosity after emptying the same by elevation. Immediate compression is applied and patient is made to walk briskly. Compression is maintained for 3 weeks.

Complications: Drug reaction and allergy, hyperpigmentation, cutaneous necrosis, infection, thrombophlebitis, rarely deep vein thrombosis.

Foam sclerotherapy: This is a new technique in which by churning in two syringes foam is formed using small quantity of sclerosant and it is injected under USG guidance to stop short of SFJ. Advancing sclerosant in varicose veins is seen clearly under USG. Minimum amount of drug is required and better contact of foam bubbles with vein wall produces better occlusion. This is the preferred therapy these days as occlusion occurs in 81% cases and tributary varicosities disappear in 96% cases.

Contraindication to Sclerotherapy

- Immobile patient
- Presence of uncontrolled malignancy
- Acute thrombophlebitis
- Peripheral arterial disease
- Hypersensitivity to sclerosant
- Associated DVT

Ablation with Radiofrequency Current or Laser Therapy

This is endovenous treatment. Under USG guidance course of varicose veins is marked. Using about 500 ml saline with local anesthesias, tumescence is produced along the course of GSV in thigh and upper leg. After puncturing dilated vein below knee, guidewire is introduced, track dilated and radiofrequency catheter or Laser fiber is inserted within the sheath. It is pushed till it is 1.5 cm distal to SFJ as judged by USG. Limb is elevated, veins emptied. Then current is fired and catheter/fiber is gradually withdrawn. Burning and collapse of the varicosity can be seen on USG. After the procedure compression stocking is applied. Electrocoagulation of the vein wall produces total loss of architecture. The procedure is comfortable for the patient and can be carried out on outpatient basis.

Some of the problems with this technique are that gross SFJ reflux, very much dilated varicose veins may be difficult to obliterate and recurrence is likely. In case of very tortuous veins, it may be difficult to negotiate guidewire. Hence procedure has to be abandoned. Smaller varicose veins need microfibers adding to the cost of treatment.

Summary

Varicose veins is a common clinical problem. Except for genetic basis and deep vein thrombosis other causative factors are not clearly documented. Most patients present with dull aching pain in calf which is increased on prolonged standing. Advanced cases may have dermatosclerosis, ulcer, etc. Duplex ultrasound is the best modality for diagnosis. Most patients are comfortable with compression stockings and phlebotrophic drugs. Foam sclerotherapy and RF/Laser ablation are best interventions in selected cases. In gross SFJ reflux, stripping and multiple stab avulsions give best lasting results.

Deep Vein Thrombosis:
A Brief Study

Epidemiology

It is difficult to say about the exact incidence of deep vein thrombosis, as the disease is clinically silent in majority of cases and in those subjects dying suddenly the cause is empirically labeled as pulmonary embolism, wherein the further study is required to document pulmonary embolism as cause of death for sure. In USA about 2.5 Lac cases occur per annum. There is no reason to believe that less than a million cases occur every year in India. Annual incidence between 48 and 182 per Lac population has been quoted in India. It is more common in females and affects most commonly lower limbs, less than 5% affecting other rare sites. Now as more and more cases are being diagnosed due to awareness of physicians, incidence is definitely on the rise and the previous feeling that the incidence of deep vein thrombosis is less in India is unfounded. Untreated deep vein thrombosis (DVT) has got risk of pulmonary embolism (PE) to the tune of 30-50%. Out of this 12% could be fatal. Recurrent DVT and post thrombotic syndrome are not uncommon.

Sources of Pulmonary Embolism

Any loose thrombus from peripheral deep veins can embolize to lungs. Proximal deep veins of the leg are found to be the most common source of PE. Other deep veins which can produce PE are proximal iliofemoral veins, deep pelvic veins, renal veins, IVC, right sided heart chambers and sometimes axillary vein. Severity of the PE is proportional to the size of the embolus and cardiorespiratory reserve of the subject. If a large embolus is thrown in pulmonary artery in a compromised cardiac or COPD patient, it is definitely going to be fatal. But showering of minor emboli repeatedly may produce symptoms, but is not fatal immediately.

Pathophysiology (Fig. 17.1)

Development of deep vein thrombosis appears to be multifactorial, because not all the patients with a particular risk factor develop DVT. The famous triad of Rudolph Virchow still holds true, of course with some modification. It consists

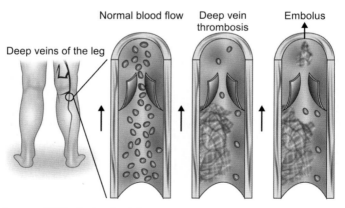

Fig. 17.1: DVT—Pathophysiology

of venous stasis, vein wall injury and hypercoagulable state. Stasis occurs due to immobilization and hypoxia of endothelial cells occurs. Stasis also decides localization of thrombosis. Normal endothelium is nonthrombogenic. However a change in the vessel wall can trigger a series of events that eventually lead to exposure of tissue necrosis factor (TNF) and activation of platelets. Prostacyclin PGI_2 also plays important role. Platelet adhesion and aggregation finally form a clot which is primarily mediated by von Willebrand Factor (vWF), a large multimetric protein present in both plasma and extracellular matrix of the subendothelial vessel wall. Thrombosis can also occur with normal vessel wall in the presence of hypercoagulable state. Normally coagulation and fibrinolysis are balanced. Imbalance between these two systems initiates thrombosis. Antithrombin III, factors VIII, V, XII, protein C and S are involved in this process. Diabetes, hypertension, hyperhomocysteinemia, dyslipidemia, sepsis all enhance this process.

Risk Factors for DVT

Depending on risk factors DVT has been divided into two types:
1. Primary DVT
2. Secondary DVT.

Primary DVT

Here the risk factors for deep venous thrombosis are not identified despite investigations. Hence it is also called "Idiopathic DVT".

Secondary DVT

Following factors are found to be associated with development of DVT.

Age

It is definitely associated with occurrence of DVT. DVT is rare in children. When the age advances from 30 to 80 years, incidence of DVT increases 30 fold. Probably advancing age induces pro-thrombotic state.

Travel

Prolonged travel has been found to be associated with increased risk of DVT, more so in older age group. This has been appreciated in passengers making long duration travel in flights in economy class in cramped position, for which airlines companies have even paid compensation. This is called "Economy Class Syndrome". Stasis could be the probable cause. Additional factors may operate.

Immobilization

This has been found to be uniformly associated with development of DVT in combination with other factors. Patients dying within 1-7 days of bed rest were studied. 15% of them were found to have associated deep vein thrombosis. In patients having stroke, incidence of DVT was 7% in normal limb, while it was 53% in the limb affected by paralysis. Hence immobilization is a definite risk- factor in causation of DVT.

Previous Thromboembolism

Previous thromboembolism makes the subject more prone for developing DVT again. About 25% patients with acute DVT have history of previous DVT. Risk of recurrent thromboembolism is higher in idiopathic DVT. Primary hypercoagulable state could be responsible for recurrent DVT.

Malignancy

It has a strong association with development of DVT, which is based on many facts. Diagnosed malignancy is present 20-30%

patients of DVT. About 15% malignancies are complicated by DVT. After diagnosis of DVT, in 5-10% patients malignancy appears within one year. Thus DVT heralds development of malignancy. These are the patients who may be initially labeled as idiopathic DVT and in due course malignancy becomes clinically manifest. Hence especially in older patients, primary DVT must be labeled with caution and relevant investigations should be carried out. Malignancy has a strong thrombogenic potential, which appears to be an important cause for this association.

Surgery

In major operations anesthesia is used which makes the patients immobile for the duration of surgery. Also as the effect of anesthesia may continue after the surgery is over, the period of immobilization is prolonged. During surgery tissue is handled, which produces tissue factor. This is responsible for inducing hypercoagulable state. In some operations like hip arthroplasty, direct manipulation around hip joint may produce endothelial injury to iliac and femoral deep veins, which could be additional factor for DVT occurrence.

Pregnancy

This has been accepted as a state of hypercoagulation. Anticoagulant factor deficiency, lupus anticoagulant, deficiency of fibrinolytic factor is reported in 20% of pregnancy related DVT. Factor V Leiden mutation (Activated protein C resistance) is an important factor in pregnancy related DVT.

Eighty to ninety-seven percent DVT occurs in left leg. Hence mechanical venous compression could be an important factor as left common iliac vein is compressed by right common iliac artery while it is crossing over. This is exaggerated by fetal head.

Trauma

Usually trauma causes immobilization. It also produces tissue injury stimulating tissue factors which induce DVT. Severe mortality and morbidity is caused in trauma cases by DVT. By venographic evaluation, incidence of DVT in injured patients is approximately less than 60%. By Duplex ultrasound incidence of DVT is about 20% which is underestimation. Age more than 40 years, blood transfusion, surgery, associated fracture of femur all these factors significantly increase DVT incidence.

Primary Hypercoagulable State

Thrombophilia syndrome, which causes hypercoagulation is an important cause for lower extremity DVT in more than 45% patients. Deficiency of Antithrombin III protein S, protein C, resistance to activated protein C (APC), hyperhomocysteinemia all have been thought to be responsible for this occurrence. In hypercoagulable states thrombi can form at unusual site and upper extremity is usually not involved.

Other Risk Factors

- Oral contraceptive and hormone supplement therapy for postmenopausal syndrome contain estrogen derivative, the prolonged use of which definitely causes DVT. More the dose of estrogen, more is the chance of developing DVT.
- Varicose veins cause dilated tortuous superficial veins, which have stagnation of blood due to increased hydrostatic pressure. There is always a chance of developing superficial vein thrombosis due to such stasis. Once superficial vein is thrombosed, there is increased proneness for developing DVT of lower extremity.
- Central venous catheters are used these days with increasing frequency. The indications are for central venous pressure monitoring and giving important life saving drugs like in open heart surgery, for inserting lead

for permanent pacemaker implantation, for intravenous hyperelimentation, etc. Keeping this catheter for long time can cause upper limb DVT.

- Inflammatory bowel disease like ulcerative colitis has higher incidence of DVT.

Clinical Features

The clinical picture of DVT is variable. Many times it is a clinically silent disease, producing mild leg edema, which is hardly noticeable especially in a bedridden patient. Usually patient presents with mild fever, dull aching pain in the limb, edema, erythema, tenderness. Severe pain in the limb is a feature of proximal iliofemoral DVT. There may be massive edema of the limb with congestion and reddish purple hue, which is called phlegmasia cerulea dolens (Fig. 17.2). When the tense edema reduces arterial perfusion also, the limb becomes tense and pale, which is called phlegmasia alba dolens (Fig. 17.3). Peripheral pulses may be absent. Petechial hemorrhages may occur. This is a stage of critical limb ischemia and the limb loss is likely if urgent intervention is not done. Another extreme of presentation is acute massive pulmonary embolism with bad general condition where salvage of life is less likely or sudden death may occur due to PE.

Patients with chronic DVT may present with chronic edema, skin hyperpigmentation, dermatosclerosis, eczema or recurrent nonhealing ulcers, condition called 'postphlebitic syndrome' or 'post-thrombotic syndrome'.

Diagnosis

- *Thrombophilia profile:* Before patient is put on anticoagulant blood sample must be withdrawn for thrombophilia profile. In primary DVT where cause of the same is not obvious, Thrombophilia syndrome should always be

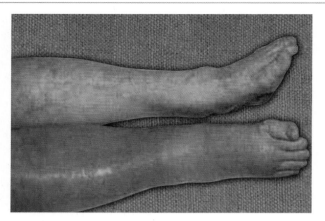

Fig. 17.2: Phlegmasia cerulea dolens

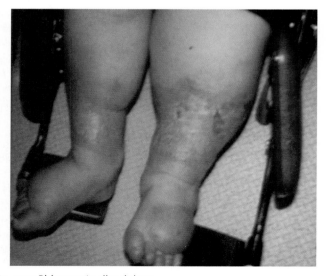

Fig. 17.3: Phlegmasia alba dolens

kept in mind as the possible cause. Deficiency of protein C and S, antithrombin III, anticardiolipin antibodies, lupus anticoagulant, hyper homocysteinemia, resistance to activated protein C (APC resistance), etc. should be evaluated.

- *D-Dimer assay:* In case of DVT occurring in any part of the body which is even clinically silent, D-dimer assay would show positive result. But if it is negative possibility of DVT is unlikely. Hence negative D-dimer almost rules out DVT.

- *Duplex ultrasound scan:* It is a very important modality to diagnose DVT. It is easily available at peripheral centers also. It can be repeated without risk to the patient, portable machine can be shifted near patient in case of emergency if the patient cannot be moved due bad general condition. Non compressible deep vein, presence of thrombus, reduced or absent blood flow in the affected vein as seen on color flow, absent phasic respiratory variation and absent augmentation on distal compression all suggest deep vein thrombosis. Being not a very costly investigation majority of the patients afford it. Some drawbacks however are inherent. It is very much operator dependent, hence expertise is necessary. It may produce false negative result and fail to image thrombi in smaller calf veins, pelvic veins and other like remote areas. But it is the investigation with maximum utility for DVT diagnosis.

- *Venography:* Using contrast is not being used commonly these days. But it is the reliable diagnostic modality with very high sensitivity and reliability, with which all other modalities are compared. It is also a research tool. DVT diagnosis missed by duplex ultrasound can be picked up by contrast Venography. But the drawbacks are that cardiac catheterization laboratory facility which is very costly, is required and the contrast dye related problems like reaction to the dye and contraindication in renally affected patients are real obstacles.

- MR venography, which does not require nephrotoxic contrast dye and can be done with the help of Gadolinium is helpful in renal failure patient also and it can image thrombi in deep veins, small veins like calf and pelvic veins. But the equipment is costly and takes time to give result.
- ^{131}I labeled fibrinogen can be detected in deep vein thrombi. But it has more or less remained a research tool.
- Ventilation perfusion scan is helpful in detecting perfusion defects in areas of lung having embolic occlusion.

Management of DVT

Why treat DVT?

The DVT most commonly occurs in deep veins of calf which has low-risk of pulmonary embolism. If left untreated, it extends to proximal deep veins in more than 20% cases. Out of these 10% have risk of fatal pulmonary embolism and about 50% have risk of recurrent DVT and nonfatal PE which could cause significant morbidity. Hence DVT must be treated.

Aims of treatment are:

- To prevent fatal pulmonary embolism (Fig. 17.4)
- To prevent recurrent DVT
- To prevent occurrence of post-thrombotic syndrome (PTS)

Post-Thrombotic Syndrome (Fig. 17.5)

Thromboprophylaxis

Main aim of treating DVT being prevention of complications as mentioned above, thromboprophylaxis must be understood clearly. The following modalities are available:

1. Graduated compression stockings.
2. Intermittent pneumatic compression.
3. Unfractionated heparin (UFH).
4. Low molecular weight heparin (LMWH).
5. Oral anticoagulants like warfarin, nicoumalone (acitrom).

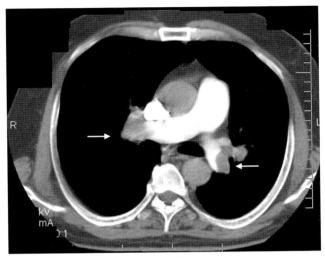

Fig. 17.4: Pulmonary angiogram showing embolus

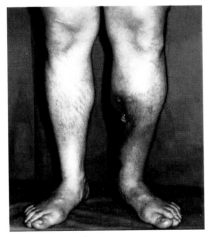

Fig. 17.5: Post-thrombotic syndrome

Graduated Compression Stockings

These are helpful to reduce venous hypertension and venous stasis and are available in different strengths like:

1. Class I—having pressure up to 18 mm Hg at ankle
2. Class II—having 18-25 mm Hg pressure at ankle
3. Class III—having 25-35 mm Hg pressure at ankle.

This is a simple, safe and moderately effective method. It is effective in preventing DVT in nearly 68% of general abdominal and gynecological operations. It is helpful in preventing occurrence of post-thrombotic syndrome. But whether it is effective in preventing fatal pulmonary embolism is not sure. The stockings are available in less allergic cotton fabric and in different colors for better cosmetic appearance.

Intermittent Pneumatic Compression (Fig. 17.6)

Pneumatic cuffs are tied at different levels in leg and thigh and are inflated in sequence from distal to proximal level producing enhanced blood flow in deep veins of leg. This

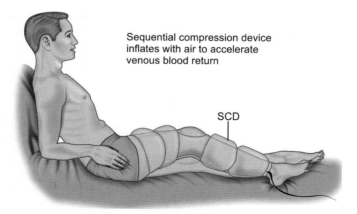

Sequential compression device inflates with air to accelerate venous blood return

SCD

Fig. 17.6: Intermittent pneumatic compression

maneuver may have antithrombotic property. It has virtually no side effects and is a valuable alternative in patients having contraindication to anticoagulant therapy. It can be given on outdoor basis.

But it is not effective in proximal iliofemoral DVT and is contraindicated in patients having peripheral arterial disease.

Unfractionated Heparin

The UFH binds to ATIII and potentiates inhibition of thrombin and factor Xa by ATIII. It also binds to plasma and platelet proteins, thereby reduces platelet function. It increases vascular permeability. It can be used in pregnancy and is cost-effective. It can be given by subcutaneous, intravenous injection and also as infusion or bolus. It is monitored by aPTT and heparin blood levels. Its side effects are bleeding complication due to platelet depletion, local hematoma and discoloration and osteoporosis if administered on long-term basis.

Low Molecular Weight Heparin

Molecular weight of LMWH is 4-5kD vs. 10-16 kD of UFH. Its bioavailability is more than 90% after subcutaneous injection. It inactivates platelet bound factor Xa. It has got less effect on platelet function and vascular permeability. Hence, hemorrhagic complications are less. It has prolonged halflife. It does not cross placental barrier, hence safe in pregnancy. Various types of LMWH available are dalteparin, nadroparin, tinzaparin, enoxaparin, etc.

Fondaparinux (Arixtra): It is a new synthetic pentasaccharide which is highly selective factor Xa inhibitor. Being synthetic it produces less reaction or allergy. It has high affinity for ATIII. It does not affect other coagulation proteins and also does not affect platelet function. Its halflife being 17 hours once daily dose is adequate.

Oral Anticoagulants

Oral anticoagulants belong to groups like warfarin, indane, nicoumalone (acitrom). They are highly water-soluble, hence their bioavailability is high. They are highly protein bound. The halflife is 36-42 hours and peak absorption period is 90 minutes. They inhibit vitamin K dependent carboxylation of factors II, VII, IX, X, protein C and S. Aspirin, NSAID, etc. enhance their effect. The dose of oral anticoagulants is monitored by INR and therapeutic range is 2-3. Major complication is bleeding, which can be controlled by vitamin K and fresh frozen plasma.

Risk Stratification of Operated Patients

The patients have been divided into three categories:
1. *Low risk:* Patients below 40 years of age, having no other risk factor and who have undergone uncomplicated abdominal or thoracic surgery fall into this category.
2. *Moderate risk:* This includes patients above 40 years of age, who have undergone abdominal or thoracic surgery lasting more than 30 minutes.
3. *High risk:* This group includes patients having history of recent thromboembolism, having undergone major abdominal/thoracic operation or major lower extremity orthopedic surgery on hip or knee joint.

Management

- *Low-risk operated patients' group:* Need early ambulation. No anticoagulants or heparin is required. Role of compression stockings is empirical.
- *Moderate-risk patients*: This generally includes neurosurgical operations, general abdominal, gynecological, thoracic operations. Prophylaxis is started 2 hours preoperatively and 12 hours postoperatively. The UFH 5000 units subcutaneous BID or injection enoxaparin 40 mg once

daily/injection. Fondaparinux 2.5 mg OD subcutaneously is given for nearly 5 days or till patient is ambulatory. Early ambulation is encouraged. If risk of bleeding is anticipated for some reason, intermittent pneumatic compression is advised.

- *High-risk group*: This includes mostly major lower limb orthopedic procedures. In hip fracture patients fixed dose LMWH like injection. Fondaparinux 2.5 mg or injection. Enoxaparin 40 mg daily is started before operation. If time is available for effective action even oral anticoagulant can be started. In polytrauma patients who are very prone to develop DVT, LMWH is the prophylaxis of choice. Prophylactic IVC filter is considered in some cases. In acute spinal cord injury with paralysis LMWH is most effective and UFH plus oral anticoagulants are less effective. Prophylaxis is continued till patient is fully mobilized or in case of paralysis till the limb is regularly exercised by physiotherapy.

Medical Patients

Patients suffering from medical disorders also need thromboprophylaxis. Low-risk patients are better with intermittent pneumatic compression. Moderate risk patients, e.g. having acute myocardial infarction and no other comorbidity are given LMWH followed by oral anticoagulants. High-risk patients like those having CCF, pneumonitis, acute respiratory failure are given low dose UHF or LMWH, e.g. injection enoxaparin 40 mg daily for 6-14 days. The protection is maintained for nearly 3 months with this.

Treatment Modalities

Thrombolytic Therapy

About 90% patients of iliofemoral DVT treated with anticoagulants alone have ambulatory venous hypertension and are prone for developing post-thrombotic syndrome, which is a morbid condition. Hence reduction of thrombus burden and early restoration of luminal patency is essential. This can be achieved by intrathrombus thrombolysis by a catheter which delivers thrombolytic agent like urokinase, reteplase, rTPA, etc. This therapy apart from restoring luminal patency, is supposed to preserve venous valves. But long duration of therapy and bleeding complications are major drawbacks.

IVC Filter

It is a device placed in inferior vena cava to prevent massive pulmonary embolism which could be fatal. One is naturally looking for ideal IVC filter which should have following features:
It should be safe and easy to insert percutaneously. It should be biocompatible, mechanically stable and nonferromagnetic, i.e. should not cause artefacts on MRI. Greenfield filter is the most commonly used IVC filter.

Indications

It is indicated when there is massive proximal iliofemoral DVT and patient has contraindication to anticoagulant therapy. Recurrent pulmonary embolism despite adequate anticoagulation and poly- trauma patient are other indications. Retrievable filters are also available now for short-term use. But follow-up of 1-2 years shows higher recurrence rate of DVT and tendency for the thrombus to form on proximal aspect of the filter. It is expensive and expertise is required.

Thrombectomy

Aim of thrombectomy is to reduce thrombus burden and to achieve early luminal patency due to which recovery occurs and incidence of post-thrombotic syndrome is reduced. This can be done in two ways:
i. *Mechanical thrombectomy:* Devices are available which can be introduces percutaneously to reach the thrombus site. The thrombus is then extracted by fragmenting and

extracting by suction. Additional thrombolysis with urokinase or any other suitable or available drug is done to take care of nonextractable thrombi.

ii. *Surgical thrombectomy:* It is rarely done these days and for specific indications as follows:

- Young patient with active lifestyle and longevity
- Contraindication to anticoagulant
- Failure of access or inadequate lysis
- Impending venous gangrene
- Proximal massive iliofemoral DVT.

The procedure is done using special venous embolectomy catheters. Additional thrombolysis has definite advantage. Sometimes in delayed cases fasciotomy is required. Though this operation is supposed to preserve valve function, recurrence rate is marginally less. Additional A-V fistula is to be created to prevent early rethrombosis.

Summary

- DVT/ VTE is a silent killer
- Treatment is mandatory to prevent fatal pulmonary embolism/post-thrombotic syndrome/recurrent DVT
- UFH/LMWH/oral anticoagulants are available for prophylaxis and treatment
- Catheter-based thrombolysis/mechanical or surgical thrombectomy can reduce thrombus burden
- IVC filter is used in limited indications
- Average duration of oral anticoagulant is 3-6 months, could be life long in some situations.

Lymphedema

About two-thirds of the body is composed of water and most of the liquid volume is contained within the cells. Remainder of the fluid is in extracellular space, which is reach in proteins and macromolecules. This fluid is called lymph. It is circulated by lymphatic system by complex mechanism. Obstruction to this lymph flow or its reflux causes lymphedema. This disorder affects about 100 million people worldwide.

Lymphedema is a progressive swelling of the extremities which is usually painless and occurs as a result of decreased lymph transport towards central veins. Developmental abnormalities like aplasia, hypoplasia, with valvular incompetence within lymphatics can be the cause for lymphedema. It may also be caused by obstruction of lymphatic flow, congenital or acquired, hampering the lymph transport.

Pathophysiology

Lymph vessels originate as blind ended sacs in the vicinity of blood capillaries which transport excess water, proteins, macromolecules, cellular elements and antigens via two sets of systems—Superficial and deep. The deep system includes organs, vessels and tissues. There are two main lymphatic channels:

1. Right lymphatic duct drains head, neck, right upper quadrant and drains into right subclavian vein.
2. Thoracic duct collects lymph from left upper quadrant, torso and both lower limbs. It drains into left internal jugular and subclavian vein junction.

Lymphatic system is a low pressure system, which is normally not fully distended or primed with lymph. Normal flow of lymph is 1.5-2.5 L in 24 hours or approximately 1-2 ml per minute. Intermittent spontaneous contractions of the axial or main lymphatic channel propel the lymph when lymphatic is distended. Propulsion is aided by muscular contractions, bowel peristalsis, inspiration, massage, etc. When the lymphatic transport is affected more than 80%, edema occurs, which remains subclinical for number of years. Cause for such event is usually occlusion of lymphatics and lymph nodes. Occasionally, lymphangiectasia with valvular incompetence and consequent lymph reflux is responsible for edema. Due to high oncotic pressure (proteins > 1.5 gm/dl) more fluid accumulates in subcutaneous tissue and skin with more proteins and macromolecules resulting in chronic lymphedema. Overlying skin becomes thick and indurated. It may show hyperkeratinization and verrucose warty projections. Skin becomes prone for developing cracks and infection leading to recurrent cellulitis and lymphangiitis. Lymphorrhea may occur through the cracks. These features produce typical clinical picture of chronic lymphedema. Edema is pitting initially. Gradually due to destruction of elastic tissue and replacement with fibrosclerotic tissue brawny edema occurs.

Etiological Classification of Lymphedema

There are basic two types of lymphedema:
1. Primary lymphedema.
2. Secondary lymphedema.

Primary Lymphedema

It is congenital or hereditary condition occurring due to aplasia, hypoplasia or hyperplasia of lymphatics. It dominantly occurs in females with ratio of 10:1 and with ratio of legs to arms of 10:1. It affects about 2 million people worldwide. Following subtypes are recognized:

A. *Congenital onset occurring before 1 year of age:* (10-25% of primary lymphedema cases)
   I. Nonfamilial
   II. Familial: It is called Milroy's disease and accounts for about 2% of primary lymphedema cases.
B. *Lymphedema praecox:* It is the most common type of primary lymphedema accounting for 65-80% of cases and occurring between 1 and 35 years of age, most often arising at puberty. Females are affected four fold more than males and one limb is involved in >70% cases. It is again of two types:
   I. Nonfamilial
   II. Familial called Meige's disease.
C. *Lymphedema tarda:* The onset occurs after the age of 35 years and is the rarest form of primary lymphedema.

Secondary Lymphedema

It occurs secondary to many causes as below:
i. Filariasis
ii. Block dissection of lymph nodes (Figs 18.1A and B)
iii. Radiation
iv. Trauma
v. Miscellaneous causes.

Filariasis is the most common cause of secondary lymphedema worldwide caused by the parasite *Wuchereria bancrofti* and *Brugia malayi* (Fig. 18.2).

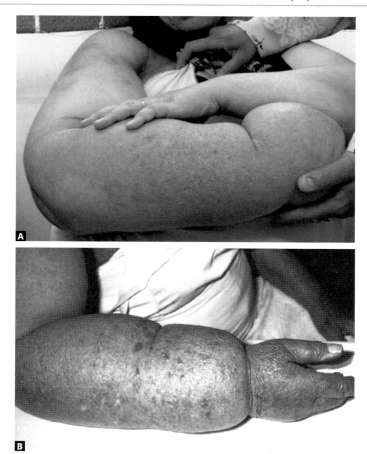

Figs 18.1A and B: Lymphedema upper limb

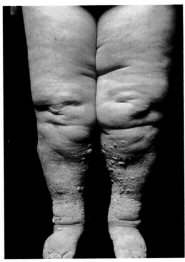

Fig. 18.2: Lymphedema lower limb

Miscellaneous causes include vein stripping surgery, burn scar excision, lipectomy, etc.

Clinical Stages of Lymphedema

There are three clinical stages of lymphedema, which are helpful for clinical categorization and for planning management, which are as follows:

Grade I: Clinically mild edema present which is pitting and reduces on limb elevation completely.

Grade II: Edema does not reduce completely on elevation, slight pitting may occur on deep pressure only, skin is thickened and fibrotic.

Grade III: No pitting, skin and subcutaneous tissue thick, fibrotic, hyperkeratosis and warty projections present.

Clinical Features

History

Family history may be positive. Teenage girl presenting with leg edema without identifiable cause indicates primary lymphedema. There may be history of discharge of milky fluid from skin vesicles suggestive of reflux. In secondary lymphedema cause may be identifiable, e.g. history of radiation and lymph node dissection surgery, trauma, presence of tumor or infection. But whether the cause is primary or secondary, the clinical presentation is similar.

Pain

Feeling of heaviness or dull ache in leg is frequently experienced but severe pain is not a feature of lymphedema. It may occur due to infection, neuritic pain in the scar tissue or after radiation.

Edema

It is usually slowly progressive. It is initially mild and pitting and gradually becomes non-pitting over number of years. It typically starts in perimalleolar area. Dorsum of foot may show typical buffalo hump. Toes become square shaped (Stemmer's sign).

Skin Changes

Initially skin looks hypervascular and pinkish. In chronic lymphedema skin becomes indurated, hyperkeratotic. Peau d' orange appearance may occur due to congestion, dilatation of dermal lymphatics. Eczematoid changes are seen in some cases. Skin vesicles may drain milky fluid. In primary lymphedema nails may become yellow due to impaired lymphatic drainage.

Infection

May occur due to cracks. Loss of chyle producing malnutrition and immune deficiency both can make patient prone to develop secondary infection. Malignant change may occur making the patient more symptomatic.

Diagnosis

Clinical examination findings along with history are quite suggestive of the diagnosis of lymphedema. But in ambiguous cases, however, diagnostic evaluation is required.

Doppler Ultrasound

It is helpful in the diagnosis of chronic venous insufficiency and arteriovenous fistula, which are important causes for chronic leg edema. Associated peripheral arterial disease can also be diagnosed, which if present compression therapy is contraindicated. Normal venous system on DUS thus favors the diagnosis of chronic lymphedema.

Lymphoscintigraphy

It is performed using ^{99m}Tc labelled antimony trisulfide colloid. Some use ^{99m}Tc labelled human serum albumin which is injected in the webspace of toes in supine position for lower extremity and tracer uptake is monitored by gamma camera. Normal transit time to regional lymph node is 15-60 minutes. Early transit indicates intravenous injection, while delayed transit suggests obstruction. This study gives information about absence/presence of lymphatics, pattern of lymphatic channels, their number and size and tracer uptake in lymph node. In lymphedema, primary or secondary, the findings usually are delayed tracer transport, dermal backflow, tracer extravasation (e.g. due to lymphangiectasia), presence of large collaterals and cross over through collaterals to contralateral lymph node. This test is 92% sensitive and 100% specific for lymphedema diagnosis.

Direct Contrast Lymphangiography

This is rarely used now and is indicated in few patients who are subject for direct microvascular reconstruction and in some with lymphangiectasia and reflux. The extent and location of dilated lymphatics are best demarcated by contrast study. It is also the best study to image thoracic duct and for exact location of lymph fistulae in abdomen, pelvis and thorax. The study is done using oily contrast.

Water-soluble contrast can be used in indirect lymphangiography. But here larger lymphatics and nodes distant to the injection site are not visualized.

Computed Tomography

It cannot differentiate between subcutaneous fat from tissue fluid and is not sensitive to define cause for leg edema. It is helpful if a tumor mass is found compressing the lymphatics.

Magnetic Resonance Imaging

It is best for soft tissue imaging and can image lymph nodes in different planes. It shows honeycombing due to accumulation of tissue fluid between fat globules in subcutaneous plane. Large lymphatic channels proximal to obstruction, which are not seen on lymphoscintigraphy, are delineated by MRI. It is particularly useful for the diagnosis of vascular lesions.

Miscellaneous

Ultrasonography may be helpful to demonstrate live adult worm in scrotal filariasis.

Measurement of tissue fluid and lymph may give idea about fluid accumulation. If the contractility is not demonstrated in lymphatics, reconstruction is not planned.

Genetic study may be helpful to evaluate some hereditary syndromes and genetic mutation like Milroy's disease.

Skin biopsy and lymph node aspiration may play important role in suspected malignancy.

Differential Diagnosis

A. *Local causes:* Chronic venous insufficiency, congenital AV malformation and AV fistula, trauma, hematoma, postoperative edema after venous bypass, etc.
B. *Systemic causes:* Congestive cardiac failure, chronic renal failure, hypoproteinemia, hypothyroidism, etc.
C. *Drugs:* Like antihypertensive drugs, e.g. nifedipine, amlodipine, hydralazine, methyldopa; hormones like estrogen, progesterone and some anti-inflammatory drugs.

Management

1. Nonoperative
2. Surgical.

Nonoperative

Preventive Measures

- In primary lymphedema presenting at birth (Milroy's diseases) and at puberty (Meige's disease) genetic basis has been documented. Hence genetic study of family members and counseling for preventive and protective measures may become a part of routine practice in future.
- Secondary lymphedema due to filariasis is the commonest form in tropical countries and also in rest of the world. Transmission is through the mosquito bites. Hence all preventive public health measures are advisable.

- *Malignancy:* Lymphedema is most common after surgery or radiation for breast, pelvic and prostate cancer. If possible lymph node dissection should be limited. Postoperatively preventive measures should be started early.
- Edema prevention measures like salt restriction, weight reduction, and elevation of the limb above heart level during supine position, exercises to improve lymph drainage and compression stockings, etc. all must be initiated early for lasting benefit. These measures are discussed in more details below.

Edema Reduction Therapy

Elevation of the limb 45 degrees above heart level helps to reduce limb edema in clinical grade I and II lymphedema. Minimum period is about 5 days initially. Stretching and aerobic exercises help to increase lymphatic transport and should become a part of life for lymphedema patients. *Massage* done by qualified, experienced technician is quite helpful (Fig. 18.3). The massage is gentle, started in the quadrant contralateral to the affected limb and in the proximal segment of the limb. Direction of the massage is from distal to proximal.

Low pressure elastic wrap bandages are effective in relieving edema and initially must be worn throughout 24 hours. In moderate edema, foam padding is used underneath to give extra support.

Compression pumps which use sequential inflation to drive lymph from distal to proximal direction are also being used. But prolonged therapy is required to gain edema reduction.

Graduated elastic stockings are available having different pressures at ankle and different lengths. Usually 50-60 mm Hg pressure at ankle is desirable and length should be enough to cover the affected area of the limb. Pressure below 30 mm Hg is of no benefit in lymphedema management. But in diabetic neuropathy, peripheral arterial disease, arthritis, ulcer patients

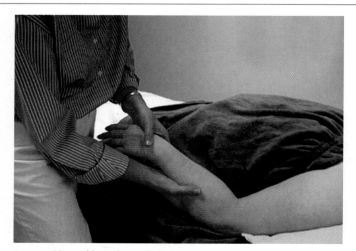

Fig. 18.3: Manual lymphatic drainage massage

modification of this therapy is required and lower pressures are accepted.

Drug Therapy

- *Diuretics:* These are used sometimes as an adjunctive therapy when edema is pitting. Short course may be given for massive edema. Long duration therapy is of no use and may be hazardous due to hemoconcentration.
- Benzopyrones (Coumarin) stimulate tissue macrophages which produces protein lysis due to which intercellular protein concentration is reduced. Consequently, edema is reduced and softening of the limb may occur. Used in the dose of 400 mg per day it is given for about 6 months and some authors have observed decrease in limb edema. But due to hepatotoxicity this drug is not used commonly.

Purified micronized flavonoids fraction (PMFF) is another benzopyrone. It is used in the dose of 500 mg twice daily for 3-6 months has shown some benefit in terms of edema reduction.

Intralymphatic steroid injection has been tried by some to decrease fibrosis. Result was unproved.

In Japan autologous lymphocytes were injected in the main artery of the affected limb in secondary lymphedema. Addition of compression therapy to this produced good benefit in short-term study.

Surgical

Aims

 i. To decrease limb size
 ii. To improve function and cosmesis
iii. To decrease recurrent cellulitis.

Absolute indication of surgery in lymphedema is suspicion of malignancy (Stewart-Treves syndrome). For other indications minimum 6 months conservative therapy must be tried before deciding in favor of surgery.

Debulking operations: These are meant to excise affected, involved skin and subcutaneous tissue to various limits.

Charles' operation: This is a circumferential excision of skin and subcutaneous tissue from tibial tuberosity to malleoli. The defect is then covered with split thickness or full thickness graft taken either from excised tissue or from normal limb. Due to high incidence of postoperative complications this procedure is seldom performed.

Miller's operation: This is a staged excision of subcutaneous tissue from medial malleolus to mid thigh. Redundant skin is excised and wound is closed with suction drain and compression stockings applied. Limb is kept elevated. This procedure has most reliable result, but must be performed only in really suitable cases as complications like infection, delayed wound healing, scarring, sensory loss and residual edema are frequently seen.

Liposuction: It is a recent modality performed through small incisions wherein subcutaneous tissue is sucked out. Results seem encouraging but are being evaluated currently.

Reconstructive procedures: Anastomosis of lymphatic to lymphatic or lymphatic to vein is done using microsurgical technique with 11-0 interrupted sutures. The procedure is expected to improve lymphatic drainage. Results are being evaluated as occlusion rate is high. Patients with secondary lymphedema of recent onset without previous episodes of cellulitis or lymphangitis are potential candidates for reconstruction.

Other procedures like buried dermal flaps, omental transposition, etc. have been tried sporadically to increase lymph flow dynamics.

Index

Page numbers followed by *f* refer to figure

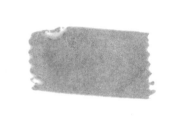